PTELEA TRIFOLIATA.

BY E. M. HALE, M.D., OF CHICAGO.

THE Ptelea trifoliata, of *Linnæus*, is a shrub or small tree of the natural order Rutaceæ; or, according to earlier views, of an order Xanthoxylaceæ, or, still earlier, of the artificial class Monœcia and order Tetra-pentandria, of the Sexual System of Linnæus.

It is figured as follows:—

Miller, Icones, t. 211;

Gærtner, de Fructibus et Seminibus, pl. 49;

Schkuhr, Botanisches Handbuch, pl. 25;

Guimpel, Fremden Holzarten, pl. 74;

La Marck, Planches de Botanique de l'Encyclopédie, pl. 84;

Duhamel, Arbres et Arbustes en Pleine Terre, 2*d ed.*, vol. 1, pl. 57;

Dictionnaire des Sciences Naturelles, pl. 128;

Mémoires du Muséum d'Histoire Naturelle, vol. 12, pl. 26;

Gray, Genera Illustrata, pl. 157;

Dillenius, Horti Elthamensis Plant. Rar., pl. 122;

Payer, Organogénie, pl. 24;

Agardh, Theoria Systematis Plantarum, pl. 19;

Loudon, Arboretum Britannicum, vol. 5, pl. 59.

The Xanthoxylaceæ included those Rutaceæ which have unisexual flowers. The genus Ptelea has polygamous flowers, with four or five stamens, with samaroid, two-celled fruit, but one-celled by abortion. Its name is the Greek for *Elm*, given because of the resemblance of the samaroid fruits.

Its six known species are all North-American. Three are Mexican,— P. pentandra, P. podocarpa, and P. angustifolia. P. mollis, of the Carolinas, is clothed with a silky pubesence. P. Baldwinii, of East Florida, has minute leaves with obtuse leaflets.

The remaining species, Ptelea trifoliata, Three-leaved Ptelea, Hop-tree, Wing-seed, Wafer-ash (known in Britain as Shrubby trefoil and Tree trefoil, in France as Orme de Samarie a trois feuilles, and in Germany as Dreiblättrige Lederblume), is indigenous throughout the United States, from the East to beyond the Mississippi, and even to Texas, in moist, shady places, and on the borders of woods and among rocks. It is a tall shrub, but under cultivation at Gordon Castle, Bannfshire, Scotland, it had, in 1835, reached the height of forty-five feet, with a trunk fifteen inches in diameter, and with branches extending twenty-seven feet from side to side.

Two varieties have been found,— one with five leaflets (P. pentaphylla, *Moench*); the other with the branches, petioles, and under surface of the leaves clothed with a soft tomentose pubescence, even when old (P. pubescens, *Pursh*).

It was originally sent to England by Bannister, but, being lost, was re-introduced by Catesby in 1724, from Carolina. It is common in the gardens of Europe; and in the Jardin des Plantes, at Paris, a tree may be seen, the crown of which had, in sixty years from planting, attained a diameter of forty-five feet.

[To this same Rue family belong the Xanthoxylum Americanum, Northern Prickly-ash, and X. Carolinianum, the Prickly-ash of the South. And in some respects they are medicinal as well as botanical analogues of the Ptelea.]

Pharmaceutical History.— The bark of the root is the officinal portion. It yields its properties to boiling water, but alcohol is the best solvent. It is, when dried, of a light brownish-yellow color externally, in cylindrical rolls or quills, a line or two in thickness, and from one to several inches in length, irregularly wrinkled and furrowed externally, with broad transverse lines or rings at short but irregular intervals, and covered with a thin epidermis; internally it is yellowish-white, but becomes darker on exposure, and is wrinkled longitudinally. It is brittle, with an almost smooth resinous fracture, granular under the microscope, resembling wax. It has a peculiar smell, which some describe as like that of liquorice root; but to me the bark, and especially the tincture, strongly resembles in odor that of the boiling linseed oil used in the manufacture of white paint. The taste is peculiar, almost indescribable: bitter, resinous, pungent, acrid, very disagreeable, speedily and powerfully acting on the mouth and fauces; and its pungency is persistent, owing probably to the oil.

The *tincture* of the bark should be made with the strongest alcohol: the addition of a small quantity of water causes it to turn as milky as the balsam of Copaiva under similar circumstances.

A *tincture-trituration* may be made from the mother-tincture, and is a very eligible preparation.

The flowers, fruit, leaves, and bark of the branches, all possess the same medicinal qualities as the root, but in a less degree. I have used the tincture of the hardly-ripe fruit. The woody portion of the shrub is but feebly medicinal. Ptelein, or the active principle, may be used in tincture, as it is perfectly soluble in alcohol; but the triturations are preferable. (See Chemical History.)

I do not know that for medicinal preparations the fresh bark possesses any superiority over the dried. The bark should be gathered in the fall,—at the time of its greatest strength,— after its constituent qualities have been fully elaborated in its cells. The leaves should be used when fully developed, but before the ripening; the flowers, just before the petals drop; and the fruits, just at the period of ripening.

The process of drying these portions should be conducted in a warm, shaded place, with care that they do not become moldy, or infested by insects of any kind.

Chemical History.—An oleo-resin, improperly called Ptelein, is considered the active principle of the Ptelea. It is described as of the consistence of thick syrup or molasses, dark-brown in mass, much lighter when in thin layers, and having a peculiar odor, somewhat similar to that of the extract of liquorice, and an oily, bitterish, acrid, persistent taste, peculiar and rather disagreeable, and acting powerfully on the fauces. It is soluble in alcohol, ether, oil of turpentine, and rather imperfectly in alkaline solutions; insoluble in acids and water. It imparts a slight milky color to water, and separates into two portions, one of which floats on the water, while the other sinks. Acetic acid added to the alcoholic or ethereal solutions does not disturb them unless added in excess. Water added to the alcoholic solution produces a milky color, precipitating the resin; added to the ethereal solution, it separates the oil, which floats on the surface. The bark was not subjected to a chemical analysis until 1862, when Geo. M. Smyser, of Philadelphia, presented an Inaugural Essay to the Philadelphia College of Pharmacy, having for its subject Ptelea trifoliata. The following were the experiments:—

"*First.* A cold infusion was prepared by percolating six drachms of the powdered leaves with water, until six ounces of liquid had passed. This was of a dark-brown color, had a bitter, aromatic taste, and an odor strongly resembling that of hops. To a portion of this infusion a solution of bichloride of mercury was added, which produced a dirty-white precipitate. And, with successive portions of the infusion, sulphuric and muriatic acids produced each a precipitate. The infusion was also coagulated by heat, showing the presence of vegetable albumen.

To a portion of the infusion a few drops of tincture of chloride of iron was added, which produced a black color. To different portions were added nitrate of silver, sulphate of copper, and a solution of gelatine, all of which produced precipitates, indicating the presence of tannic acid. The portion which was precipitated by gelatine was filtered; and, with the filtered liquid, tincture of chloride of iron produced a greenish-black color, which disappeared when the liquid was heated, showing the presence of gallic acid.

"*Second.* An infusion of the fruit was prepared, similar to that from the leaves. This infusion had a very bitter taste, and, upon treating it as in the former experiments, the result was the same.

"*Third.* Two and a half ounces of the powdered fruit was treated with ether,—to deprive it of fixed oil,—dried and treated with alcohol. To the resulting tincture, acetate of lead was added, which threw down a large quantity of coloring matter and some resin: the liquid was filtered, and treated by passing sulphureted hydrogen through it to get rid of the excess of lead, and then again filtered and heated to drive off the excess of sulphureted hydrogen. To the liquid, yet warm, water was added in drops until it began to produce a precipitate. It was then placed on a sand-bath, and evaporated to a syrupy consistence: when it had cooled, it was agitated with an equal bulk of chloroform; and, when allowed to rest a few minutes, it separated into two layers, the watery liquid being on the top; this was decanted, and on evaporation yielded a small quantity of an extract of a very bitter taste. I made repeated attempts to obtain crystals from this extract, but without success. The chloroformic solution, when evaporated, gave a soft, resinous substance of a slightly acrid, bitter taste.

"*Fourth.* Three ounces of the powdered fruit was moistened with equal parts of alcohol and water, placed in a percolator, and the menstruum of alcohol and water passed through it until it was exhausted. The resulting tincture was evaporated to an extract, which was of a dark-brown color and a bitter, acrid taste. One drachm of this extract was washed with alcohol, which dissolved out a small quantity of a soft resin, which was very acrid to the taste. The same part of the extract was washed with ether; this dissolved a portion of it, and on evaporation yielded a brittle resin, which was odorless and almost tasteless. The part which remained after being washed with the alcohol and ether was principally bitter, extractive matter, and which had none of the acrimony of the extract."

MEDICAL HISTORY. — The first mention of the Ptelea in the medical literature of this country is found in Rafinesque's Medical Botany. He observes that "the leaves are vulnerary, used for poultices, good for worms." In Louisiana "it is called Bois-puant." He makes no mention of the bark of the root. It is mentioned in Griffith's Medical Botany: "The native species P. trifoliata, is said by Schœpf to be anthelmintic, for which purpose the leaves and young shoots are used in strong infusion. The fruit is aromatic and bitter, and is stated to be a good substitute for hops."

In Howard's Botanic Medicine, 1836, it is described under the vulgar names of Heal-all, Ague-bark, Pickaway, Anise, and Wing-seed. "The bark of the root is an excellent stimulant, expectorant, tonic; useful in all cases of debility, and particularly in agues. It has been highly extolled as a remedy in consumption of the lungs, having been sold as a nostrum at a high price. In this instance it was tinctured in whiskey."

In Dr. J. G. Jones's Eclectic Practice (first edition), it was erroneously mentioned under the name of Staphylea trifolia, the name of another shrub in no way resembling it. In the second edition it was properly designated as Ptelea trifoliata, and extolled as "a pure, unirritating tonic, having rather a soothing influence when applied to irritated mucous membranes." He advises it "in the convalescence after fevers, and in debility connected with gastro-enteritic irritation. It promotes the appetite, enables the stomach to endure suitable nourishment, favors the early re-establishment of digestion, and will be tolerated by the stomach when other tonics are rejected." He prescribes the cold infusion, half a fluidounce every two or four hours.

In the various eclectic medical journals have appeared, from time to time, short articles alluding to its powers as a tonic. (See Eclectic Med. Jour., Cincinnati, 1867, p. 159.) King's Dispensatory describes it, and, in addition to the above medicinal uses, says: "A tincture made of Ptelea in whiskey is reputed to have cured several cases of asthma, and it is said to *cause, in many instances where it has been used, a troublesome, external erysipelatous inflammation, either general or local, but which, if the use of the tincture be persisted in, finally disappears, and the patient becomes at the same time cured of the disease for which he was treated.*"

Jones and Scudder, in their Eclectic Materia Medica (1858), add: "We have found a saturated solution of it beneficial in chronic rheumatism." They assert it to be "alterative, tonic, stomachic, diaphoretic, excitant," etc. Scudder has "known it to be employed in epilepsy with decided advantage."

Dr. Kost (Mat. Med., p. 631) has an article on Ptelea.

These crude uses and unscientific recommendations comprise all that can be gleaned from eclectic sources up to this time.

It has formed the basis of many nostrums, "ague-cures," "tonics," and even "expectorants." In 1866, Mr. Chapman, of Hudson, Michigan, manufactured a preparation of "Pepsin and Wafer-ash," in which the pepsin was united with the tincture of Ptelea, pure anhydrous glycerine being used as the menstruum. This preparation is very extensively used by some physicians as a chemico-dynamic remedy in dyspepsia, and very highly valued for its curative virtues. In my own practice, and under my observation, cases of atonic dyspepsia, with deficiency of gastric uice, have been cured by this preparation, when the usual rem

2

edies failed to effect any improvement. A notable symptom in all these cases was, profound depression of spirits.

The first homœopathic physician who used the Ptelea in any form was Dr. P. H. Hale. Guided by the pathogenetic symptom found in King's Dispensatory, he gave it in some obstinate cases of chronic erysipelatous disease; also in affections of the bronchia and stomach, arising from the metastasis of such eruptions. He made some notable cures with the lower dilutions. At the meeting of the Western Institute of Homœopathy, held at Indianapolis, in 1867, Dr. Hale reported some of these cases, but they have not yet been published. I have occasionally prescribed it for symptoms similar to those obtained in the provings, especially a variety of urticaria, in which the raised spots assumed the appearance of a bruise. In a few cases it appeared to relieve the pain and itching, and shorten the duration of the disease. I do not know of any other clinical experience in the homœopathic school.

Allopathic experience is very limited. The only report on its use is to be found in Tilden's Journal of Materia Medica, vol. 5, page 321, by Dr. O. F. Potter, of St. Louis, Mo.

History of the Provings.—In 1866, the American Institute of Homœopathy appointed me one of the Bureau of Materia Medica. I selected Ptelea as the subject of my report, and offered two prizes for the best two series of physiological provings, and one prize of $50 for the best pathological proving on animals, "to consist of all the symptoms observed during life, a record of the pathological or normal appearance of each organ after death, a microscopic examination of the diseased organ or tissue, and any abnormal tissue or product."

At the time of the annual meeting of the Institute, in 1867, I had received only four physiological provings. I did not, therefore, award any prizes, or send in any report to the Institute, except the request to be continued on the Bureau during the next year. In the course of the year 1868, I received seven additional series of physiological provings, but no pathological experiment. I name the following provers in the order of the excellence of their experiments: —

1. Prof. T. Nichol, M.D., of Belleville, (First Prize).
2. Drs. Fish and Train (Second Prize).
3. Dr. Wm. H. Burt, of Lincoln, Ill.
4. Dr. Cowles, of Bloomington, Ill.
5. Dr. A. Cowperthwait, of Toulon, Ill.
6. Dr. C. H. Lutes, of Ligonier, Ind.
7. Dr. C. W. Pierce, of Ft. Smith, Ark.
8. Dr. A. V. Marshall, of West Cornwall, Vt.
9. Dr. E. Parsons, of Kewanee, Ill.
10. Dr. Hayward, of Romeo, Mich.
11. Dr. Hunter, of Bellefontaine, O.

Total, twenty-two provings.

PROVINGS BY PROF. THOMAS NICHOL, M.D.

Prover, thirty-six years of age; strong and muscular; of sanguine temperament, with fair hair and gray eyes. Has been for a number of years accustomed to experiment with drugs, and is easily affected by them.

First Proving.

April 16, 1867. — Being in perfect health, took thirty drops of the strong tincture of Ptelea. In a few minutes, roughness of the fauces, with feeling as if vomiting would come on. At twenty minutes to nine, A.M., sudden and unexpected urging to stool. Stool at first of natural consistence, but towards the close thinner and diarrhœic, with slight tenesmus. Passage accompanied by sweat on the forehead and head, though the morning was cool. Half past nine, A.M. Slight but persistent nausea, not at all disagreeable, somewhat resembling the effect of a few inhalations of sulphuric ether. Pressive feeling at the base of the brain, with nausea, closely resembling the well-known Ipecac symptom: "Headache, as if the hair and skull were bruised, penetrating through the bones down to the root of the tongue, with nausea." Flushes of heat, alternating with chilliness, all through the day. Pulse 88. The appetite good at dinner, but entirely absent at supper-time. At five, P.M., urging to stool, at an unusual time. Half past six, P M., stool, with straining; the discharge thinner than usual. Slight, but persistent nausea from nine till eleven, P.M.

April 17, quarter past seven, A M.—Thirty drops. Sleep during the preceding night restless; languid and unrefreshed on waking. Feverish heat, lasting all day, accompanied by pains in all the limbs, and nausea. Disinclination for mental exertion. Frontal headache all day, pressing from within outwards.

April 18, noon.—Forty drops; immediately followed by retching, with increase of the frontal headache. At quarter to one, P.M., piercing pain shooting through the temples, with increased headache and nausea. After dinner, increased nausea, with heat of skin and profuse perspiration on the forehead; pulse 96, small and hard. Half past one, P.M. Inclination to vomit gradually passing off. In the evening, amelioration of all the symptoms; though still languid and drowsy. Constipation; no morning stool as usual, but at seven, P.M., small, hard stool, after much straining. Sound sleep all night, but haunted by frightful dreams.

April 19.—The symptoms were an exact copy of those developed on the preceding day.

Four, P.M.—Forty drops. Resolved to let this dose act for twenty-four hours, and then go on with more frequent doses.

April 20.—Awakened at one, A.M., by a pressing pain in the stomach; a feeling as of a weight; worse on motion, and aggravated by pressure with the hands. Also a rising of bitter fluid, with a deathly nausea, confusion of the head, and sweat on the forehead. Thoughts chased each other through the mind, it seeming impossible to fix the attention upon any one object.

This attack, which resembled acute dyspepsia, lasted from one till five, A.M., followed by sleep until seven, A.M.; languid and tired on awaking. During the whole forenoon, sharp pains in the right hypochondriac region

Half past three, P.M.—Twenty drops in water. At four, P.M., had sour risings from the stomach; heat of skin; pulse 96, small and fluttering. Nausea all the afternoon and evening, with splitting headache, incapacitating for mental exertion.

April 21, half past ten, A.M.—Thirty drops. Extraordinary inclination to sleep. Bitter taste in the mouth; the tongue, which had hitherto been clean, was coated with a yellowish fur, and the nausea was persistent. No stool to-day (an unusual occurrence). Up to this date, the medicine had had no effect on the temper, but to-day it produced fretfulness and irritability without the slightest exciting cause. Sleepiness excessive; went to bed at eight, P.M. At a quarter past nine, was roused to go and see a patient, and on awaking was attacked with a kind of nightmare; quite conscious, but unable to stir on account of a pressing weight in the stomach and whole front of the trunk.

April 22.—On rising, giddiness, with piercing pain through the brain, accompanied by severe aching pain in the stomach.

Quarter past six, A.M.—Thirty drops. All day, from six, A.M., till three, P.M., urging to stool, with rumbling in the bowels.

Three, P.M.—Thirty drops. The sickness of the stomach less to-day.

April 23, half past seven, A.M.—Thirty drops. Hard and difficult stool, with smarting of the anus after the passage. Three, P.M. Tenderness of the splenic region, with soreness to the touch.

Four, P.M.—Thirty drops. Giddiness, with vertigo at five, P.M.; vertigo long-continued, and, after it, increase of abdominal tenderness.

April 24, seven, A.M.—Forty drops. The abdominal pain extending more toward the umbilical region, and worse on motion. On drawing a long breath, a sharp stitch proceeds from the umbilicus, toward the back-bone, and the tenderness on pressure is increased. Half past eleven, A.M. Sharp, cutting pains through the front of the brain, alleviated by pressing it with the hands. Three, P.M. — Forty drops.

April 25. — Sleep last night restless and uneasy, awaking unrefreshed and languid. The abdomen much swollen, and tender over its whole extent, especially over the splenic region.

Six, A.M. — Forty drops. Nine, A.M. Hard and difficult stool.

Ten, A.M. — Forty drops. Persistent nausea and vomiting, with giddiness of the head, and a feeling as if unsteady in the legs. Unfit for mental exertion all day, and toward the afternoon had to give up exertion of every kind.

Five, P.M. — Forty drops, and again at ten.

April 26, half past six, A.M. — Fifty drops. The giddiness of head and reeling in walking much increased.

Three, P.M. — Fifty drops. Four, P.M. The pain in the splenic region much increased, and the swelling evidently greater. Constant feeling of weight in the hypochondria when walking: a dragging pain, which affects the right as well as the left side.

Six, P.M. — Fifty drops. Head confused and giddy when retiring to bed, at half past ten.

April 27. — Head weak and confused. Seven, A.M. — Fifty drops. Nine, A.M. Attacked with too much giddiness and vertigo to keep up. Nausea and vomiting soon followed, although no relief came after the vomiting; bitter taste in the mouth; tongue dry and coated brownish-yellow; splenic pain much aggravated. Hot and feverish all day.

I was obliged to discontinue the proving, as the effects were so severe. I have had attacks before, but nothing of such a bilious character. I insert the symptoms for the reasons given by Dr. Dudgeon, on page 209 of Lectures on the Theory and Practice of Homœopathy: "He (the prover) should be in a good state of health, — not necessarily absolutely healthy, for that is a rare property. He may possess what is called an idiosyncrasy, a weak point, and yet be perfectly capable of physiological experimentation, and the symptoms developed in him by virtue of this idiosyncrasy may still be received as part of the action of the medicine; for what is this idiosyncrasy but a tendency to be acted on by a specific with more than usual severity? It is in fact only the predisposing cause heightened in sensitiveness; and for the action of the medicine, as well as of the morbific agent, a predisposing cause is always requisite."

Second Proving.

Oct. 21, 1867, quarter to seven, A.M. — Ten drops of tincture. Half past seven, A.M. Slight nausea rising from the stomach upwards, accompanied by roughness of the back part of the tongue. A very mild nausea — by no means unpleasant — lasted during the whole forenoon.

Eleven, A.M. — Fifteen drops. At dinner the appetite not as good as usual, though, before beginning the proving, it had been keen. Throughout the course of the meal, the same faint nausea persisted. One, P.M. Aching pain at the base of the brain, though the intellectual powers were as active as usual. At four, P.M., ate a bunch of somewhat tart grapes, and all the symptoms disappeared; the nausea and headache were entirely removed in a few minutes.

Quarter past eight, P.M. — Twenty drops. At half past nine, nausea, with rumbling in the bowels, accompanied by discharge of flatus, with desire for stool. Nausea, and pressing pain in the forehead; the pain presses from within outwards. No passage from the bowels to day, — a very unusual occurrence. At eleven, P.M., went to bed. Nausea aggravated by lying down. Restless and tossing, and some difficulty in falling asleep.

Oct. 22. — The dreams during the night were so vivid and lifelike as to seem, on waking, as if he had been up all night. In the morning, weak and languid; hands and feet hot and feverish; pulse 72, weak and fluttering.

Half past six, A.M. — Twenty-five drops. At half past seven, ringing in the ears, with slight giddiness, the ringing lasting from two to three minutes, and returning for the same length of time half an hour later. Little appetite for breakfast; the bread seemed tasteless; no thirst. Quarter past nine, A.M. Transient giddiness, with heat of the head and face, especially on the forehead. Goes about his professional duties in a perfunctory manner, very unlike the fiery zeal with which he usually combats disease and his allopathic step-brethren. Heaviness in the occipital region, with gloomy feeling in the forehead. At dinner, all food seemed tasteless. Three, P.M. Faint feeling in the stomach, with sourish rising. The nausea is much worse on walking. At quarter to seven P.M., was weighing out a trituration, and the mental confusion was so great that he had some difficulty in telling what was the tenth part of 150 grains. Appetite, at ten, was indifferently good, but food was still tasteless. Singing increases the nausea, and aggravates the headache, causing shooting pains from within outwards. At quarter past eight, P.M., a squeezing pain in the epigastric region.

Half past nine, P.M. — Twenty-five drops. In bed, the griping pain in the epigastric region worse than during the day, and the abdomen swollen, but not painful. During the night, heavy sleep, with less vivid dreams than on the previous night. Frontal headache, so severe that he almost felt it during sleep; and, on waking at intervals during the night, noted that it was more intense than during the day.

Oct. 23. — The heavy, pressing, frontal headache still continues; the pain pressing from within outwards, aggravated by stooping. Less nausea; stomach now feels weak. Aching pains with occasional stitching in the region of the diaphragm.

Twenty minutes past seven, A.M. — Twenty-five drops. At Eight, A M., regurgitation, tasting of the medicine, but with little nausea. Temper as good as usual yesterday, but to-day was unusually annoyed by noise. Headache, a stunning, pressing pain in the frontal region, closely resembling a chronic headache, which he had had for many years, and which his master in the institutes of homœopathy, Dr. Constantine Hering cured with one prescription of Rhus toxicodendron. At dinner, a complete repugnance to animal food, although there was less nausea than on the preceding day. Unable to eat rich pudding, of which he is ordinarily fond. At two, P.M., head languid and heavy; unable to follow the train of thought when reading what is by no means difficult. Strong inclination to lie down and rest. At ten minutes past two, sour risings from the stomach, with feeling of weight and uneasiness in the stomach. Half past eight, P.M. His intellectual powers moved slowly and heavily, and had difficulty in recalling familiar things to mind. At ten minutes past nine, P.M., slight vertigo, with a choking feeling in the pharynx. Took no dose, at noon or night, to-day. All the afternoon, felt a curious *malaise*, which prevented him from doing business with alacrity. Attended to his duties as usual, but felt such an oppression and weakness at the stomach that he had no heart to work. Stools, to-day and yesterday, of usual consistence and slimy coating.

Oct. 24. — The sleep during the preceding night was heavy but restless, with fantastic dreams, — practising medicine among people of gigantic stature; suddenly the scene would change, and his patients were about the size of peas. When awake, during the night, felt that the weight at the stomach was much worse than during the day. Conscious of the stunning headache before he was awake. Extraordinary weakness of memory; was unable to recall the names of familiar people. Felt feverish, irritable, and intolerant of noise. At breakfast he ate some pudding; symptoms all aggravated at once, especially the heaviness at the stomach and the difficulty of concentrating thought. One, P.M. At dinner, complete disgust at animal food, — unable to eat any, — and the appetite was very poor. Quarter past three, P.M. Eructations, tasting of rotten eggs. Dry heat over the whole body, especially in the palms of the hands; pulse 104, small and weak. Aching, pressive pain in the temples, aggravated by chewing. Aching pains in the back part of the thighs. At four, P.M., hard stool, with straining. Soon after, eructations, almost bringing on emesis. Half past four, P.M. Aching in the bowels while walking; on standing still; pain aggravated by a deep inspiration; severe prostration of mind. At ten, P.M., a sharp, cutting pain in the right hypochondriac region, aggravated by deep inspiration, sufficiently severe to prevent sleep.

Oct. 25. — Sleep heavy and dream-haunted. Quarter to seven, A.M — Five drops. Splitting headache, aggravated by stooping, moving the eyes, and by reading. Dull, heavy pain in the right hypochondriac region, apparently on the convex surface of the liver. No passage from the bowels. At dinner, ate roast beef and pudding. Pain and distress in the stomach soon after, with feeling as if a stone were there.

Five, P.M. — Ten drops. Throbbing pain in the epigastric region, aggravated by full and deep respiration. Urine is deeper in color, and scalds slightly during passage. Weakness of mind very marked. Sleep good.

Oct. 26. — Sleep was better last night; awoke with the usual morning headache, with weight at the stomach. Aching of all the limbs, especially of the flexor muscles. Half past seven, A.M. Fifteen drops. At quarter to twelve, A.M., griping pains, with rumbling in the right iliac fossa. The epigastric region is sore to the touch, and pressure aggravates the nausea. Two, P.M. Pain and soreness extending from the right to the left hypochondriac regions, but worse in the epigastric region; a feeling of weight, aggravated by standing erect or sitting erect, and relieved by stooping forward. Good appetite at dinner, but the usual aggravation followed. Urine was high-colored, — the "yellowish-red" of Neubauer and Vogel. At supper, voracious appetite, followed by pain in the epigastric region; despondency. Slight swelling in the region of the liver.

Ten, P.M. — Twenty drops.

Oct. 27. — Sleep uneasy and unrefreshing, and with more annoying dreams than before. Awoke with dry heat over the whole body, especially on the face and hands. The tongue was coated yellow, and the papillæ were red and prominent. Bitter taste in the mouth, with dryness.

Quarter to nine. — Twenty drops. This morning the headache is so severe that mental exertion is a burden, and the pain is materially aggravated by any attempt at study. The face is yellowish, and the skin feels dry and harsh. The dry heat over the body continues, though the feet are cold. The appetite is now voracious; food has not its natural taste; and pain at the stomach follows every meal. The liver is perceptibly swollen, and sore on pressure, which causes a dull and aching pain.

Nov. 1. — Has taken none of the drug since Oct. 27. The effects mentioned in the proving have gradually declined. The only new phase consists in a number of thoracic symptoms, which have come on very gradually, and which now cause considerable pain. As the various gastric and hepatic symptoms declined, uneasiness and difficulty in breathing came on, with dull pain, especially in the right infra-clavicular region, accompanied by hacking cough without expectoration. This has come on very insidiously, and now the right lung is dull on percussion, especially in the right infra-clavicular region. On auscultating the region over the bifurcation of the trachea and the upper part of the sternum (with Cammann's stethoscope), the respiration was found to be tubular, the sound was higher in pitch than the normal vesicular sound, and more rapidly evolved. Expiration and inspiration were of equal length, with a slight interval between them. On making a full inspiration, sharp pains shot from the sternum towards the nipples, especially that of the left side. Pressure on the intercostal spaces close to the sternum caused pain of a dull, aching nature. These thoracic symptoms were better in the house, and aggravated by exposure to the keen air.

Nov. 7. — The thoracic symptoms had gradually declined.

Third Proving.

November 29, 1867, half past seven, A.M. — Took twenty drops sixth dec. dil. Ate a light breakfast at a quarter to eight. Weight and fullness at the stomach in an hour afterwards, with dull headache, pressing from within outwards. The headache does not incapacitate for mental exertion, but causes a languor and indisposition to work. At twenty minutes past eleven, A.M., griping in the stomach, with sharp pain on slight pressure. At dinner appetite very poor, after driving in the cool air all the forenoon. Twenty minutes past two, P.M. Rumbling in the umbilical region, with swelling accompanied by slight vertigo, with sweat on the forehead. At three, P.M., eructations of a bitter taste, with slight nausea. Marked indisposition for mental work. Ten minutes past three. Straining at stool, with increase of the vertigo. Twenty-five minutes past three, P.M. Increase of the headache, with marked forgetfulness. In writing a letter, felt a curious and unusual disposition to hurry through with it as quickly as possible, hardly taking time to write the words. The headache and vertigo were aggravated by even a moderate warmth of the room; all the symptoms aggravated in a hot room, and ameliorated in the cool air.

Quarter to nine, P.M. Twenty drops. At nine, P.M., involuntary discharge of flatus, with urging to stool.

November 30. —Sleep unusually deep and heavy. Racking frontal headache on waking, aggravated by rolling the eyes upward. Weight in the stomach, with bloating of the abdomen.

Continued speaking, even for five minutes, causes stitching pains in the diaphragm.

Half past seven, A.M. — Twenty drops sixth decimal dilution. At quarter to eleven, A.M., the headache had been persistent; sharp pains shoot from the right to the left frontal region. At ten minutes before noon, eructations, with a bitter taste in the mouth, causing nausea and abortive attempts at vomiting. At dinner, marked repugnance to butter and fatty foods. A very moderate meal was followed in half an hour by a sensation of stuffing and fullness. Headache a little better before dinner; an hour and a half after, much worse, and aggravated by mental exertion. Stitching pains in the upper part of the posterior mediastinum, aggravated by deep breathing, and by the recumbent position; this is accompanied by soreness of the trapezius muscles. Forgetfulness is even more marked than yesterday. The headache worse. Half past three, P.M. An attack of vertigo, without any exciting cause, other than the Ptelea. Attack so violent as to compel discontinuance of writing and to bow the head on the hands, closing the eyes. The vertigo was preceded and accompanied by mild nausea, with slight griping pains in the stomach. During the attack the pains in the posterior mediastinum were aggravated. At seven, P.M., urging to stool, but it merely resulted in the difficult discharge of a few balls of hardened fæces. During the whole day, unusual indisposition to mental or physical exertion.

Half past nine, P.M. — Twenty drops.

Dec. 1.—Sleep broken and restless; and, at waking intervals, hardly able to determine whether sleeping or waking. Unpleasant dreams during the whole night. Awoke at seven, A.M., languid and unrefreshed.

Eight, A.M. — Twenty drops. At half past eight, dull aching pains in the left scapula, aggravated by the slight exertion of writing. Ten minutes to nine, A.M. Griping pain in the epigastrium, aggravated by speaking and by deep respiration; pressure aggravates the pain. and causes nausea. *Malaise* of body and mind; desire to lie on the lounge, and "think of nothing at all." Drowsy and sleepy during the whole afternoon, with bitter taste in the mouth. At five, P.M., urging to stool; a continued pressure on the rectum, but on attempting to have passage it resulted in nothing.

Ten minutes to ten, P.M. — Twenty drops.

Dec. 2.—Sleep broken by dreams, at first of a frightful nature, but, towards morning, lascivious. Awoke languid and unrefreshed, and with the feeling of being mentally unequal to the business of the day.

Seven, A.M. — Twenty drops. After breakfast, ineffectual urging to stool, as on the previous day. Lassitude and weariness, with disposition to hurry. At three, P.M., feeling of weight, and dull pain in the right hypochondriac region, with qualmishness of the stomach. The feeling of pressure in the rectum lasted all day, and, at five, finally resulted in the discharge of a small quantity of indurated fæces, with only slight relief. There is, apparently, a true torpor of the rectum.

Nine, P.M. — Twenty drops.

Dec. 3. — Awoke at six, with a bruised sensation in all the limbs, especially worse in the muscles of the back. The sore, bruised pain was increased by pressure with the fingers.

Eight, A.M. — Twenty drops. Hot, dry feeling, over the whole body, with a sensation as of having slept without undressing, or having sat up all night. The tongue coated yellowish, with red papillæ; bitter taste in the mouth, with absence of thirst. Appetite deficient, and food has an unnatural taste, as on recovering from a long illness. Mental lassitude, as on the previous day. The right hypochondriac region is swollen, and the clothes feel too tight. Irritable mood; a very slight annoyance keeps recurring to his mind, impelling him to speak about it. Better able to study than on previous day, but difficult to concentrate his thoughts. More forgetful than before the proving; and yet, by collecting the thoughts, able to recall things read many years ago. Able to supply some additional items to a professional paper, intended to be exhaustive. At four, P.M., the lumbar pains, aggravated, with stitching pains in the right hypochondriac region, which is swollen. At half-past six, P.M., racking frontal headache, with heat of the face and head. Able to examine patients, but inclined to hurry through with it; and, in selecting the remedy, inclined to follow Fred Humphrey's rule, — "First impressions are the best." The appetite good at supper; pressure on the stomach, and increase of the hepatic pains after a light meal.

Quarter past ten. — Twenty drops. No stool today, but continual urging in the rectum.

Dec. 4.—Awake nearly all night from the harassing nature of the pains, especially in the back, — in all the regions, but especially the dorsal. Dry heat; most on the parts where the pain is worst. The hepatic pain is aggravated, also the urging in the rectum. At breakfast, repugnance to butter; even a small quantity aggravates the epigastric pain.

Three, P.M.— Twenty drops. All the symptoms are aggravated in the warm room and ameliorated in the open air. The muscular pains are relieved by rapid motion in the open air, though they are worse on commencing motion. Rumbling in the bowels, with tenderness on pressure.

Dec. 5.—Awoke by the pains in the back; less in the limbs than on the preceding day. The pain accompanied by rumbling in the bowels, with bloating and tenderness on pressure. Liver feels heavy and sore, especially when lying on the left side. Less pressure on the rectum than formerly. The mental lassitude and forgetfulness continue. At supper, ate some sour apple-sauce, when all the symptoms became milder and gradually disappeared. During the whole experiment, the urine was redder than usual.

Fourth Proving.

Dec. 13, 1867, twenty-five minutes past noon.—Being in excellent health, a little before dinner-time, took, five hundred drops of the concentrated tincture. Before taking the dose, had a good appetite, but, after swallowing it, found that he could not bear the sight or smell of food, especially of roast beef. Rumbling in the stomach, with inclination to vomit. Chilliness and shivering over the whole body; could not keep warm, even by sitting over the stove. Confusion of thought, with hurriedness of manner. Forgetfulness,— writing one familiar word for another of similar sound. Pulse quickened from 72 to 104 in fifteen minutes; small and hard. At quarter to one, P.M., on turning the head to look at the clock, taken with sudden giddiness and with faint feeling. Sick and faint, with a sudden shrinking from any mental work. At five minutes to one, P.M., the taste of the medicine continually returning in gusts to the mouth; a feeling as if vomiting would relieve. Turning the head, even gradually, aggravated the vertigo. At one, P.M., pressure over the eyes, aggravated by lifting the eyebrows. Sudden sleepiness. Five minutes later, too giddy to sit up. Ordinary conversation in the room greatly annoys. Ten minutes past one, P.M. The qualmishness increased, and the old pressure at the rectum returned. Rising from the chair aggravated the vertigo; the frontal headache was aggravated by moving the eyes, and by noise; speaking aggravated the nausea. Shivering in a warm room, and the head hot; shivering from the hips downwards. Rising aggravates the giddiness, and also the nausea. Burning and qualmishness at the stomach, with pain on pressure. Attempting to walk aggravates the vertigo very much; unable to stand alone.

Eructations, tasting of the medicine, with increased nausea; bitterness in the mouth, with dryness. Twenty-six minutes past one, P.M. The pain in the head, the nausea, and the pressure in the rectum aggravated by rising. A little ordinary writing, difficult, from vertigo and confusion of mind. Thirty-five minutes past one. Pulse 126, small and thready; shivering, with chattering of the teeth, scarcely comfortable near a large fire. Ten minutes past two. All the symptoms ameliorated by a walk in the open air. Half-past two, P.M. Aching, drawing pains in the left ankle, aggravated by motion; the pain extends up the calf of the leg. Dryness of the mouth, with bitter taste. Drawing pain in the left elbow. Ten minutes later. Extreme forgetfulness. Quarter to three, P.M. Violent urging to stool. Three, P.M. Stool of more fluid consistence than usual, and of very fetid smell; followed by renewed urging in the rectum. The passage is accompanied by chilliness and shivering. Twenty-five minutes past three, P.M. Marked dryness of the lips and tongue, with hawking of mucus from the pharynx. Sickly paleness of the face, especially around the eyes. Languid and dull, with little inclination for either mental or physical exertion.

Quarter to four, P.M. Shuddering and horripilation, with eructations tasting of Ptelea. At Four, P.M., a griping, contractive pain in the stomach for half an hour. Half-past four. The pain moved downwards to the abdomen. Quarter to five. Urging to stool, and sudden discharge of a quantity of thin diarrhœic fæces, of cadaverous smell, with smarting of the anus. Rumbling in the bowels after stool. Five, P.M. Rending pains around the left knee, which come and go rapidly. Very little appetite, after eleven hours' abstinence, with a strong repugnance to butter. Twenty minutes past seven, P.M. Another stool of the same nature as the previous one, yet somewhat thinner in consistence, and even more cadaverous in smell. Lassitude of mind, with disinclination to study; tasks performed in a perfunctory manner. Thirty-five minutes past eight, P.M. Griping in the bowels, with swelling of the liver, which is tender to pressure.

Retired at nine. Very sick indeed. After a restless, dream-

4

haunted slumber till one, A.M., awoke with a seated, dull, heavy pain in the abdominal region, felt distinctly in the liver, which was easiest when lying on the right side; also a feeling of pressure on the lungs, and of suffocation when lying on the back. Lying on the left side, the liver dragging on its ligaments, and swollen and tender even to a light touch. There is also griping in the bowels, with rumbling, and pressure in the rectum. Abdomen bloated; pressure increased the griping. Rending, tearing pains in the left scapula. Head hot and feverish, with dull aching in the frontal region, especially on moving the eyes. Dry heat over the whole body, especially on the palms of the hands. Restless and uneasy; unable to sleep. At half past five, A.M., fell into a light sleep, and awoke at seven, tired and unrefreshed.

Dec. 14.—Bitter taste in the mouth; tongue dry and coated, light brown. Appetite at breakfast poor, with the usual repugnance to butter. Eating a very small piece of cheese aggravated all the hepatic and gastric symptoms. All the symptoms are better in the open air, though rapid motion causes sharp pains in the right hypochondriac and epigastric regions. The griping and rumbling continue, and there is pressure on the rectum, such as precedes a dysenteric passage. Urine scanty, and of a deep reddish-yellow tint. Labor performed in a perfunctory manner. Mind feels dazed and languid.

Quarter past eight, A.M.—A discharge of fæces, coated with slime. The passage is followed by tenesmus, which brings on a small discharge of fæces with a larger quantity of mucus, and this again is followed by tenesmus. During the stool, shuddering with chilliness of the sacral region; after the stool, smarting of the anus, with itching. The dejection does not relieve the pressure of the rectum, which becomes worse as night advances. Half past ten, P.M. The pulse at 104, very small and weak. Eleven, P.M. A sudden attack of vertigo, lasting about one minute. Quarter past eleven, P.M. Great dryness of the mouth.

Dec. 15. — Slept from midnight till about seven, A.M. The pain in the forehead is deeper in the brain than it has been. Pressure, as of a stone at the pit of the stomach, aggravated by a light meal. Dry heat over the body, with sweat on the forehead. Eleven, A.M. A dull, aching pain in the small of the back, aggravated by motion. Thirty-five minutes past eleven, A.M. Acute, cutting pain in the spleen. Forty minutes past two, P.M. Aching, drawing pains in the left scapula and shoulder-joint. Ten, P.M. All day had felt extremely weak. Remembered having heard Dr. Constantine Hering in his famous morning lectures, which, with characteristic kindliness, were without money and without price, lay down the position that "*provers generally indulge in superlatives.*" Nevertheless, felt entirely justified in writing "extremely weak." Felt weak in every limb, — weak in brain, weak in memory, thought, and will, as if a powerful and all-pervading disease had fastened upon him.

Dec. 16. — Slept all night, though the sleep was dream-haunted, as before. Became conscious of a dull, aching pain in the small of the back; motion adds a sharp, sticking pain to the dull one. Heavy, aching pain in the liver, with deficient appetite. Half past eleven, A.M. Copious stool of fluid consistence and bilious smell, with a very copious expulsion of ascarides. Stool followed by tenesmus, and succeeded by itching and smarting of the anus. Had to work a good deal to-day, though weak in body and mind.

Dec. 17. — Slept from ten, P.M., till four, when he was awakened by the severity of the lumbar pain, worse than yesterday morning. Weight and pain in the liver relieved by lying on the right side; aggravated by lying on the left, which causes a dragging pain. Griping in the epigastric region, with dryness of the mouth, yellow-coated tongue, and bitter taste. Weak and irritable all the forenoon, and with the frontal headache incessant through the proving. Legs weak during the forenoon, with drawing pains in the knees and the flexor muscles.

Dec. 18. — One long and remarkably vivid dream all night, till four. Awakened by hepatic and gastric symptoms, all of which are aggravated towards morning. The urine, all through the proving, of deep reddish-yellow, and small in quantity. No stool all day. Appetite better than on former days.

Dec. 19. — Last night sat up till half past eleven, with a view of testing whether the early waking was a result of the remedy, or a mere accident. Was very sleepy when he went to bed, but, nevertheless, awoke about half past three. The gastric and hepatic symptoms were milder than they had been. Forty minutes past seven. A stool of natural consistence, smell, and appearance. Appetite at breakfast very poor, with muddled feeling in the head. Ten, P.M. All the symptoms have declined to-day, especially the headache.

PROVINGS BY DRS. FISH AND TRAIN.

Prover, twenty-five years old, with nervo-sanguineous temperament; light hair, blue eyes, and light build; weight one hundred and thirty-five pounds; in excellent health, having been free from sickness of any serious character for years; appetite good; diet temperate, using coffee once a day; continued the same during the proving as before; never used intoxicating liquors in any shape, nor tobacco.

First Proving.

March 30, 1867, ten, A.M. — Took ten drops of the tincture. Soon experienced a sensation of nausea, with a nervous pain alternating from the left arm to left eye and parietal region.

Noon. — Ten drops. Dinner in half an hour, followed by an empty feeling in the stomach.

Two, P.M. — Fifteen drops. Great lassitude and weariness throughout the afternoon. Unusual fatigue after slight exertion.

Half past six, P.M. — Twenty drops. Nausea for a few minutes. In about an hour began to be feverish, thirsty, lips cracked and sore, — an unusual occurrence with the prover. Slept soundly during the night. Saliva very profuse; ran from the mouth during sleep, and wet the pillow.

March 31, four, A.M. — Awoke (earlier than customary) with some fever, accelerated pulse, parched mouth, and an awakening of sexual desire. Took no medicine during the forenoon. Slight, continuous headache, lowness of spirits.

Two, P.M. — Twenty drops one hour after a hearty meal. Felt a burden in the stomach soon after, although previously no discomfort was produced by the dinner. It all passed away in two hours. Four, P.M. Felt very well; some lassitude.

Six, P.M. — Thirty drops. Within ten minutes, a full, throbbing headache, with dizziness and nausea; radial pulse, 68, but very strong, so as to be readily seen. Headache continued the same for half an hour, when it became sharp, and darted from temple to temple; very painful, especially when moving. Urinated five ounces (two ounces more than normal quantity). Natural in appearance; no evidence of albumen or urea crystals by tests. At seven, P.M., pain in the hypogastrium, in the region of the bladder; continued fifteen minutes. During this time the headache intermitted. Headache resumed in the left zygomatic region. These aches are very changeable, shooting rather quickly from place to place. Dull pain sets in about eight, P.M., in the umbilical region, quite severe, continuing half an hour. All symptoms disappeared during the evening.

Half past nine, P.M. — Thirty drops. Urinated five and a half ounces; clear. Retired soon after, and slept soundly during the night.

April 1, five, A.M. — Awoke refreshed; saliva flowed from mouth very profusely during the night; sexual desire increased; flatulence. Pulse slow, strong, irregular, 60; urinated six ounces; normal in appearance.

Six, P.M. — Twenty drops. Slight return of the head symptoms. In half an hour, full, pressive ache in the frontal and temporal regions.

Eleven, A.M. — Thirty drops. Stool, natural; headache, oppression at the epigastrium; unsteadiness and nervous irritability.

Half past one, P.M. — Thirty drops. Rumbling in the bowels; constriction of the pharynx; painful sensations in the temporal region, continuing over an hour. During the afternoon, a sensation of languor and weariness spreads over the whole system.

Six, P.M. — Thirty drops. Dull, oppressive headache came on while reading, about nine. Urinated six ounces; rumbling in the bowels; perceptible increase in the flow of saliva. Retired at ten. Slept well, with the exception of troublesome driveling.

April 2. — Awoke about six, A.M. Took no medicine during the forenoon. Very languid; energy entirely gone. Appetite normal; urinated seven ounces. Stool natural; borborygmus; considerable flighty headache. Took ten drops at three, P.M., at fifteen minutes past, at half past, at four, and at half past. The attendant symptoms were headache, oppression, pain in the stomach, evident signs of gastralgia, tenderness at the sternum, and sensitiveness to the light during the whole day.

Five, P.M. — Twenty drops. Slight nausea; pulse full and hard, very irregular; feeling as of sand in the stomach; urinated six and a half ounces, clear, normal. Retired at nine with the usual feeling of *malaise;* head just ready to ache. Slept unusually well; saliva not so troublesome.

April 3, six, A.M. — Awoke with desire to urinate; passed seven ounces, clear. Unusual hunger, craving for acid food. Twenty drops. Headache in the frontal and temporal regions.

Eleven, A.M. — Twenty drops. Headache; weariness; urinated seven and a half ounces. Two, P.M. Headache in the occipital region, lasting half an hour, passing then to the frontal, over the eyes, not very severe. Six, P.M. — Twenty drops.

Passed seven ounces clear urine, natural stool. At ten, P.M. urinated five and a half ounces. Uneasiness in the bowels, with flatulence; unusual quantity of saliva, thin and watery. Retired at quarter past ten. Sleep disturbed by dreams. Driveling.

April 4, six, A.M. — Awoke feeling much refreshed; no pains or aches; urinated nine ounces. Took no medicine during the day. The day passed with scarcely a recurrence of symptoms till evening, when the feeling of uneasiness in the bowels (umbilical region) came on, increasing in severity until nine, when it was almost intolerable. It was of a peculiar character, bearing down, sometimes spasmodic, and griping; sometimes sharp and throbbing. Ten, P.M. Some relief, but a headache set in, confined to the temporal regions. Urinated seven and a half ounces. This really severe attack passed off by midnight, and sleep brought entire relief.

April 5, half past five, A.M. — Awoke with the same pain in the bowels as the night before. Appetite poor; ate a light breakfast, which seemed to afford some relief.

Nine, A.M. — Twenty drops. At quarter past ten, pain in the bowels came on with redoubled vigor; headache also set in; obliged to lie down; great increase in the amount of saliva; urinated eight ounces. One, P.M. Pain less; headache less; appetite pretty good; ate a light dinner. Two, P.M. No pain for an hour and a half. Three, P.M. A slight touch in the umbilical region, disappearing in half an hour. Drowsiness succeeded, and the slightest effort seemed to weary. Five, P.M. But little change; no prominent symptoms. Retired at half past ten. Urinated during the evening eight and a half ounces; stool natural.

April 6. — Slight headache in the morning. No trouble in the stomach or bowels until after dinner, when, immediately after eating, the stomach seemed perfectly empty; very troublesome sensation of goneness. Somewhat feverish; pulse natural, rather full. During the preceding days the fever-symptoms had been absent. Some headache during the evening. Urinated during the day twenty-five ounces. Stool natural.

April 7, half past five, A.M.—Headache set in upon waking; continued during the forenoon. Pulse 85, full. Feverish; thirsty, with a dry feeling all over the system. Voided twenty-seven ounces of rather clear urine. No further symptoms.

April 8.—No symptoms during the entire day, except the same nervous weakness of the eyes, experienced during the early part of the proving. Whole system seems relieved. Urinated twenty-two and a half ounces. Pulse natural; stool natural.

April 9.—Slight headache in the morning. Feels perfectly well.

During the above proving, the appetite was generally good, the bowels natural; respiration unchanged; pulse, first full and hard, but, during the severe symptoms, quiet; again feverish and full at the close. Urine greatly increased in quantity, in quality unchanged. Saliva very abundant; almost constant driveling during sleep.

Second Proving.

April 16, 1867.—One week from the last record of the first proving. During the past few days the prover has felt unusually well.

Seven, A.M.—Forty drops of tincture. Slight nausea.

One, P.M.—Forty drops. Quick, sudden starts of headache during the afternoon; *malaise.*

Seven, P.M.—Forty drops. A general change in the system seemed to have taken place, and the former weary feeling supervened, with tenderness of the abdominal viscera,—i.e., readiness to become painful. Retired at ten. Felt a strange uneasiness in the bladder and prostate. Smarting sensation in the urethra upon urinating, rising out of bed for the purpose. Nearly ten ounces were passed. Smarting in urethra continued for twenty minutes after urinating.

April 17, morning. — Felt well. Eight, A.M. — Sixty drops. An immediate feeling of heaviness in the stomach; eructation of wind; nausea; felt well in an hour.

Ten, A.M. — Sixty drops. Repetition of former symptoms. Well again an hour after.

Three, P.M. — Sixty drops. Headache now set in. At about five, the old pain in the umbilical region became a prominent symptom. The headache and pain continued without intermission; both rather severe.

Ten, P.M. — Took sixty drops and retired. Passed a restless night. Arose twice to urinate. Passed during the day and night thirty-one ounces. Stool natural.

April 18, five, A.M. — Arose, feeling sore, tired, and sick. Headache soon set in. Urinated nine ounces.

Eight, A.M. —Sixty drops. Appetite not very good. Umbilical region very tender, and seemingly on the point of aching. Noon, ate a light dinner. Urinated eight and a half ounces.

One, P.M. — Sixty drops. During the afternoon noticed an increase in the amount of saliva. Spitting became frequent, though unusual in health. Headache severe.

Three, P.M. — Sixty drops. Pain in the umbilicus and stomach set in with vigor. Throbbing headache in the frontal and temporal regions; very painful. Pain in the abdomen, very severe. Nervous irritability of the eyes. Urinated six ounces. Stool natural.

Seven, P.M.—Feeling very sick. Took sixty drops, and retired. Restless, and in pain all over the head, stomach, and bladder. At eight, was obliged to get up and urinate; passed six and a half ounces. Considerable burning in the urethra. Heat in the region of the prostate. Pulse full, hard, tense, but not rapid. Skin dry and parched; lips cracked, although the saliva is greatly increased in quantity, and keeps up a constant driveling while lying on the face. Rolled around till after midnight, when sleep gave some intermission to the constant pain.

April 19, nine, A.M. — Arose with headache, feeling very sore, tired, and disgusted with everything. Urinated about six ounces. Pulse more rapid (90). Took one hundred drops, followed in an hour by thirty-five more. Nothing experienced from the fresh doses until about half past eleven, when, on a sudden movement, the headache became violent, and the whole abdominal region began to ache and pain. Rumbling in the bowels, followed at half past twelve by a diarrhœic stool, very dark in color, and sulphurous in smell. Pulse much more natural than on the preceding day. Saliva very abundant. Appetite all gone; eyes sensitive to light; general *malaise*. Pain in the bowels was eased but a moment by the stool. Three, P.M. Symptoms unchanged. Half past four. Headache confined to the left side. Abdominal pain settled to a steady, dull pain, not so severe as before. Diarrhœic stool. Headache passed off after the stool. Abdominal pain the same. Six, P.M. Headache resumed. Relieved at nine, feeling better than the night before, yet in much pain. Urine not measured during the day; about the same in amount as the day before; saliva not very troublesome.

April 20. — Same general feeling of *malaise*, tenderness and pain in the umbilicus, and dull headache continued all day. Slept most of the afternoon. Three stools during the day, rather diarrhœic; urine nearer the normal amount; pulse rapid, — from 80 to 90; saliva troublesome.

April 21. — Occasional headache; bowel pains continue. Stools diarrhœic. Diarrhœic stools continued a full week, when the unnatural condition was removed. In a week more, the tendency to headache had passed off, but it was full three weeks before pressure on the abdomen could be endured without pain.

An unusual amount of saliva has troubled the prover ever since. Urine natural in a few days.

THIRD PROVING.

Prover, twenty-one years of age; nervo-sanguineous temperament; light-brown hair; gray eyes; weight, one hundred and twenty-five pounds; in good health; no constitutional disease; temperate in habits, never indulging in the use of ardent spirits or tobacco. The medicine was of the third dilution, prepared with distilled water by the decimal scale, from Prof. Hale's tincture. Diet unchanged during proving.

April 15, 1867, seven, A.M. — Took five drops. No symptoms. At eleven, took five drops. No symptoms. At six, P.M., five drops. Tickling in urethra after urinating. Urine deposits muddy sediment.

April 16, seven, A.M. — Ten drops; dull headache set in at about ten.

Half past eleven. — Ten drops. At two, P.M, urine increased in amount, filled with whitish sediment. Sensitiveness of the urethra; headache continues.

Six, P.M. — Ten drops. Feeling of nausea; pulse rapid at bedtime; oppressive headache over eyes.

April 17, seven, A.M. — Fifteen drops. No symptoms during forenoon. Fifteen drops at half past eleven. Headache during afternoon; soreness at pit of stomach; appetite poor.

Six, P.M. — Fifteen drops. Headache increases during evening; quite severe upon retiring. Urine more nearly normal.

April 18, six, AM. — Arose feeling restless and uneasy. Sleep disturbed by dreams. Perceptible increase in sexual desire. Awoke during night with nightmare.

Seven, A.M. — Took fifteen drops. No special symptoms during forenoon. Took fif een drops at half past eleven; pulse, small and rapid; thirst; furred tongue; poor appetite; desire for acid food; headache; nervousness.

Six, P.M., fifteen drops. Diarrhœic stool; headache continued; drank a great deal of water; retired at nine, feeling unwell.

April 19, seven, A.M. — Took fifteen drops. Repetition of symptoms of day before; diarrhœa; five stools during the day.

Half past eleven.—Fifteen drops. Headache during afternoon; feverish.

Six, P.M. — Fifteen drops. Felt better during the evening; urine, normal.

April 20, seven, A.M. — Slept much better than night before. Took fifteen drops. Headache; some diarrhœa; no further symptoms during day, with the exception of a diarrhœic stool and feeling of *malaise.*

April 21. — Awoke with slight headache, which passed off during the forenoon; diarrhœa; urine increased in quantity; pulse natural.

April 22. — No symptoms.

The diarrhœa passed off in the course of a few days, and no further effects were experienced from the proving.

PROVINGS BY WM. H. BURT, M.D.

Prover of sanguine-nervous temperament, with a little of the lymphatic; weight, one hundred and forty-eight pounds; habits temperate, using no form of distilled or spirituous liquors, tobacco, coffee, or the like. Health excellent; appetite good; bowels move regularly once a day, generally in the morning.

First Proving.

April 20, 1867, six, A.M. — Took half an ounce of thirtieth dec. dil., prepared by myself in rain-water. Had a natural stool before breakfast. At ten, A.M., had a stool of a mushy character, with distress in the hypogastric region. At noon, dull, pressive pains in the temples, with occasional fine, neuralgic pains in the temples. The headache is aggravated by walking. Headache continued all day, with eructations of sour fluid from the stomach, and great lowness of spirits. A sour stomach is something he is never troubled with.

April 21.— Great depression of spirits all day, with a black, lumpy stool at two, P.M.

April 22, six, A.M.—Took half an ounce one hour before eating. Felt unusually well all day until eight, P.M.; then had colicky pains in the small intestines every few minutes for one hour; the pains were not severe.

April 23, five, A.M.—Mushy stool; another at ten, P.M. Unusually irritable all day, with slight, colicky pain in the epigastric region, and drawing distress in right hypochondrium. Legs ached all day.

April 24, six, A.M.—Half an ounce. Had a few sharp pains in the arms in the morning. While in bed in the evening, had fine, prickly pains in the fingers.

Second Proving.

The thirtieth dilution produced so few symptoms upon him, that he determined to use the sixth, prepared as before, in rain-water.

April 27, six, A.M.—Feeling well. Took half an ounce an hour before eating. At half past six, severe distress in the region of the spleen. Seven. Sudden, pressive pain in the temples; it feels as if the temples would be pressed together; with distress in the epigastric region. Eight. Natural stool, followed by distress in the anus. Nine, A.M. Constant distress in the small intestines, with an urgency to stool. Occasional flying pains in the abdomen. Dull, frontal headache, feeling as if the temples would be pressed together. Drawing pains in the left heel. Noon. Have had frequent distress in the bowels. Two, P.M. Had severe nausea for five minutes, with distress in the umbilicus, and dull, pressive headache. Frequent fine pains in the fingers, and region of the spleen. Nine, P.M. Languid all day, with aching distress in all the joints, especially in the knees, ankles, and feet. All the evening had a drawing, aching distress in the right hypochondrium.

April 28, seven, A.M. — Half an ounce, half an hour before breakfast. A number of times through the forenoon had a feeling in the forehead as if it was being pressed together from temple to temple, with severe distress in the region of the spleen and right side of umbilicus; stool rather constipated. Very languid all the afternoon, with severe, aching distress in the wrists, knees, ankles, and feet. Fine, sharp pains in the fingers. Dull, aching distress in the small of the back. Constant aching distress in the whole abdomen. The pressive headache has troubled me more than any other symptom to-day, with the aching in the back and legs.

April 29. — Awoke with severe backache, which passed off in one hour. Seven, A.M. — Half an ounce, an hour before eating. Several times through the forenoon had pressive pains from one temple to the other; natural stool. Very languid from noon until six, with flushed face and a feeling as if I had fever; but the pulse was two beats below the natural standard. Constant frontal headache, with severe pressive pains in the temples, from one temple to the other, every ten or fifteen minutes. Almost constant cutting pains in the left umbilical and epigastric region, with aching distress in the right hypochondrium. Frequent rumbling in the bowels, with desire for stool. Dull backache.

April 30. — Awoke with severe pain in lumbar region.

Seven, A.M. — Half an ounce, one hour before eating. Had constant pressive headache, with aching distress in the bowels, back and legs, with great languor, all the forenoon. Natural stool. Head, back, knees, and calves of the legs continued aching severely all day, with rheumatic drawing pains in the elbows and bowels. Fauces feel sore. Atmosphere quite damp.

May 1, 1867. — Languid all day, with aching distress in the small of the back, knees, and calves of the legs. A number of times through the day had hard, pressive pains in the temples.

Very irritable and desponding. Natural stool. Frequent drawing pains in the right and left hypochondrium. Occasional sharp pains in the stomach.

May 2. — Legs and back ached all the afternoon. Several times through the day had drawing pains in right elbow-joint and fingers. Natural stool.

May 3. — Natural stool. Legs ached all the afternoon until seven, P.M.

THIRD PROVING.

May 6, noon. — Feeling well. Took half an ounce of the second dec. dil., half an hour before dinner. In the afternoon, had hard, pressive pains at times in the left temple, with frequent cutting pains in the epigastric and umbilical regions, and constant drawing pains in the wrists, knees, and ankles, worse in the right knee and right wrist and fingers. Had very severe aching distress in the right knee all the evening; had repeated colicky pains in the small intestines, lasting but a minute or two at a time.

May 7. — Natural stool, morning and night, with colicky pains in the hypogastrium in the evening, before stool.

May 8, six, A.M. — Half an ounce. In the forenoon had slight distress in the abdomen, but all the afternoon had severe aching distress in the whole lumbar and sacral region. Natural stool, morning and night.

May 9. — Awoke with hard headache; passed off in a short time. Natural stool. Seven, A.M. — Half ounce of the first dec. dil. one hour before eating. At eight, A.M., sharp pains in the umbilicus. Three, P.M. Excessive languor, with a feeling as if he had fever; pulse 88, soft and weak, with constant inclination to yawn. Five, P.M. For the last hour has had colicky pains in the umbilicus, and drawing pains in the hands and ankles. Pulse 74; feeling much better. Once in the evening had hard, pressing pains in the right temple.

May 10.—Awoke with severe backache, which lasted about half an hour. Six, A.M.—Two ounces first dec. dil. one and a half hours before eating. At eight, A.M., natural stool. Several times in the forenoon had severe cutting pains in the right temple. Noon. For the last hour has had constant distress in the right hypochondrium and epigastric region, with drawing pains in the fingers and ankles. Three, P.M. Very languid and feverish; pulse 88. Has had frequent cutting pains in the umbilicus.

May 11.—Same symptoms as yesterday, but not so strongly marked.

Had a few rheumatic symptoms for several days, similar to the above noted.

Fourth Proving.

May 27, 1867, six, A.M.—Feeling well. Took forty grains of the solid extract, prepared by myself from the bark of the root of a Ptelea tree six inches in diameter. In twenty minutes, sharp neuralgic pains in the right temple. In forty minutes, dull distress in the stomach, with fine stitches in right temple. Seven, A.M. Frequent darting pains in right temple, with constant distress in stomach (probably mechanical). In one hour and ten minutes after taking the medicine, ate breakfast, which relieved the distress in the stomach. At nine, A.M., natural but lumpy stool. Same pains in the temples. Tongue feeling as if it had been scalded; the whole upper surface feels as after taking Aconite. Noon. Has had, a number of times, fine, sharp pains of a pressive character in the left temple. Tongue still has fine, sticking pains all over the upper surface. Frequent distress in the stomach. Aching distress in the calves of both legs. Hands hot and dry. Three, P.M. Feeling feverish, hands are hot and dry, and ache constantly. Pulse 80. Occasional pains in the left temple. At five, P.M., hard, dull, aching pains in the wrists, hands, fingers, and ancles. Nine, P.M. Tongue has felt as if it were scalded all day; occasional pains in the bowels. Languid feeling. Thermometer 62. Rainy day.

May 28. — Slept well; awoke very languid. Tongue coated yellow, and feeling rough. Urine high-colored. Lumpy, dark-colored stool.

Six, A.M. — Took eighty grains. Ate breakfast an hour and a quarter after. Eight, A.M. Dull headache, with a feeling as if he had fever; breath seems to burn the nostrils. Tongue feeling as if it had been burned. Nothing tastes natural. Distress in the epigastrium; had constant dull headache all the forenoon, with frequent paroxysms of pain in the right temple, as if it would be pressed to the left side. Noon. Smarting of the eyes. Acrid feeling in the tongue. Languid and feverish. Rheumatic pains in the wrist, hands, fingers, knees, and ankles. Four, P.M. Languid, with dull feeling of the head. Several times through the afternoon and evening had sharp, colicky pains in the umbilical region. Thermometer 70. Cloudy day.

May 29. — Slept well. Rough, flat taste in the mouth; tongue yellow, coated along the centre and base. Natural stool.

Six, A.M. — One hundred and fifty grains. In half an hour, hard, pressive pain in right temple. Breakfast at half past seven. Nine, A.M. Severe, dull headache, aggravated by walking upstairs. Stinging, biting sensation all over the tongue. Teeth all ache and feel sore; increased flow of saliva that tastes saltish. Hands and fingers ache constantly. Ten minutes before noon. Severe nausea for two minutes, with efforts to vomit. Has had a severe dull headache all day, aggravated by walking. Increased secretion of saliva, with biting sensation in the tongue. Burning distress in the epigastrium (not severe). Slight colicky pains in the umbilical region. Dull, aching distress in the hands, fingers, knees, and ankles. Breath seems so hot that it irritates the nostrils; pulse 74. Languid. At two, P.M., soft stool. Nine, P.M. Same symptoms as in the forenoon, but not so strongly marked.

PROVINGS BY MRS. S. M.

Under the Direction of Dr. Cowles.

Prover aged twenty-seven; of a bilious-sanguine temperament; with dark-brown, or almost black, hair and eyes; of decided, yet mild, disposition; with strong constitution. A housekeeper. General health has been regarded good. Has been troubled somewhat with sedimentous urine, after the use of some kinds of food. Some tendency to rheumatism. Requires about eight hours of sleep regularly; subject to dreams, yet sleep is good and refreshing. For some days previous to proving, found urine as follows: Variation in quantity from twenty-two to thirty-five ounces; average for fourteen days was twenty-eight ounces. When it was the least, it had some red sediment upon standing. Weather mild and pleasant. No epidemic.

First Proving.

April 6, 1867. — Took ten drops of the first dec. dil. on sugar, regularly three times a day, about one hour before eating. Ten, A.M. Feels a trembling and weariness in the lower limbs. Two, P.M. Rumbling in bowels. Four, P.M. Stitches in shoulder and hip. Nine, P.M. Dull pain in left shoulder-blade, and some unpleasant sensation in stomach; sticking pain in left knee.

April 7. — On getting up, had a feeling of lameness in small of back. Urine during last twenty-four hours only sixteen ounces, with reddish, cloudy sediment. Six, P.M. — Soon after taking the drug, had a pain behind the right ear; also twice during the evening.

April 8. — Lameness in back on getting up. Twenty ounces of clear urine. Half past eleven. About half an hour after taking drug, had a sharp pain behind the right ear, near the carotid artery. Three, P.M. Hiccough; face burns; dull pain in right side of head; pain behind right ear. From two to six, slight burning in face, followed by rheumatic pains in right leg and arm. Nine, P.M. Pain in back of left breast near the axilla; feeling rather languid; appetite somewhat increased.

April 9. — Had dreams of food and awoke hungry. Dull, rheumatic pain in anterior muscles of right femur and humerus, which disappear after getting up. Twenty-four ounces of rather red urine. Afternoon. Some pain in left biceps muscle. Six, P.M. Pain behind right ear, in left temple and in back of neck. Ten, P.M. Hard pain in left side of head, and behind right ear.

April 10. — Slept pretty well, but had some dreams of food. Awoke towards morning, feeling somewhat feverish. Awoke having hard, sticking pain in left temple, followed by a dull headache, and cords of the neck lame on the right side; occasional stitches behind the right ear; pulse 104, quick, small, and somewhat intermittent; mouth and throat dry; a faint feeling in stomach. About noon, headache, worse in left temple; pain in back of neck; whole neck feels swollen; pain in right mastoid process of temporal bone. Two, P.M. Pulse 84; head aches, and feels large. Three, P. M. Pulse 96; hot flushes and pain in top of head and eyes. For three days has had no stool till to-day. Stool nearly natural. Rainy by spells to-day. Feels sick all over and indifferent to duties. Went to bed in the afternoon and soon to sleep. Awoke at five, P.M., with pain behind right ear and in shoulder, near the spine of right scapula; a lame spot on the inside of right knee as large as a penny; otherwise quite well.

April 11. — A cool night after the rain. Had ten hours of sound, refreshing sleep. Feels quite well; pulse 80; twenty-eight ounces of clear urine in the last twenty-four hours. Lame spot still felt; back somewhat lame on waking. Eleven, A.M. A few minutes after taking drug, had a very severe pain in the right ear;

had been ironing one hour. Pulse 92. Two, P.M. Severe backache, worse in lumbar region; transient rheumatic pains in right side and right shoulder-blade; dull pain in region of liver. Had a slight headache and an unpleasant feeling in the throat all the afternoon. Five, P.M. Pulse 88, and occasionally intermitting. Seven, P.M. Feels as though diarrhœa were coming; desire for stool, tenesmus, but no stool. Heat and dryness of the œsophagus, as before.

April 12.—Slept ten hours. Awoke three or four times during the night with hard pain in the bowels; mouth and throat very dry. Awoke with backache, and unable to speak aloud for some time; a faint feeling. Twenty-one ounces of clear urine in twenty-four hours. Pulse 75. Weary feeling in the limbs; rheumatic pains in arms. Two, P.M. Pulse 106; hot flushes and slight headache. Seven, P.M. Hard backache the whole length of spine and back of neck; also through right shoulder. Appetite good, but no stool for two days.

April 13.—Had a restless night, full of dreams, with some fever. Backache in the morning, pain in the bowels, and constipation. Nine, A.M. Hard stool, and after it a smarting like piles. Some backache and shooting pains through shoulder and chest. Has taken no more of the drug since yesterday. Two, P.M. Pulse 96, with burning cheeks and hot flushes.

Symptoms passed off in three or four days after leaving off the drug. Less tendency to costiveness.

Second Proving.

May 7, 1867.—The tasks incident to a change of abode have required much more labor than usual. During the week past, has had a rather profuse flow of urine of a light color, with occasional rheumatic pains in upper and lower limbs, and neuralgic headache one afternoon, which was relieved by Aconite. Bowels regular, not having been costive since ceasing to take drug. Catamenia returned two days too soon, and quite copious.

The second experiment was with the sixth decimal attenuation. During the seven days of proving, took ten drops regularly three times a day. Weather warm and pleasant. No epidemic.

No symptoms on the first day, except a slight headache after a long walk. During evening took slight cold.

May 8. — Thirty ounces of clear urine during last twenty-four hours. Soft stool at seven, A.M. Eight, A.M. Pulse 88. Three, P.M. Pulse 82. No symptoms.

May 9. — Slept soundly all night, but dreamed of dead animals. Twenty-six ounces of clear urine in twenty-four hours. Nine, A.M. Felt a sharp pain behind the right ear; has not felt one since the last proving, and never any before that. Increasing appetite. No stool to-day.

May 10. — Slept well and feels well. Twenty-six ounces of urine in twenty four hours; pain behind the right ear at half past eight, A.M. Increasing appetite. At seven, P.M., soft stool, with tenesmus.

May 11. — Twenty-eight ounces of urine in twenty-four hours. Slept very soundly. Hungry all the time; unusual energy to work; in fact, feels better than before commencing the proving. At night had a slight headache. Retired at eight, and slept soundly all night.

May 12. — On awaking, had a pain in the small of the back, which ceased after rising, leaving, for a while, a tired feeling. Eight, A.M. Soft stool. At nine, A.M., felt a hard pain in the epigastrium, with slight feeling of nausea for about five minutes and afterwards, three or four times during the day. Bowels slightly distended at night, and feeling like diarrhœa. During the day would be startled at slight, unusual sounds. Went to bed early, and slept soundly all night.

May 13. — Feels lame in the region of the kidneys, on waking. Soon after rising and taking drug, felt sharp stitches through the right lung, which is sound. Soon after, had a pain behind the right ear, which she felt certain was caused by the drug. Bowels soon felt tendency to diarrhœa. Eight, A.M. Very soft stool. At ten, a darting pain under right breast. From two to four, P.M., headache on the left side, and sharp pain in left temple. Pulse 92.

May 14. — Awoke with headache and hunger, both of which passed off after a hearty breakfast. Urine twenty-eight ounces in twenty-four hours; clear. Took last dose in this proving this morning. Rumbling in bowels. Eight, A.M. Had a sharp pain in left ear. Two, P.M. After a walk, lay down and slept three hours. Awoke with slight pain near the heart, and afterward shooting pain under the right breast. Pulse, on rising, 100; one hour later, 80. Natural stool in the evening.

Remarks. — Thinks the provings have improved the condition of kidneys. Bowels nearly natural after first proving, but very costive since the second.

PROVINGS BY MR. ALLEN C. COWPERTHWAIT.

Prover a student of medicine. Age twenty years; mental-vital temperament predominant; dark hair; gray eyes; weighs one hundred and forty-two pounds; height five feet eight inches.

First Proving.

March 17, 1867. — Took five drops of sixth dec. dil., four times per day, — one hour before each meal, and before going to bed. Eleven, A.M. A severe frontal headache, lasting about ten minutes. One, P.M. Dull frontal headache, lasting all the afternoon.

March 18, seven, A.M. — Dull feeling, with sensation of weakness in upper extremities, which lasts all day. Towards evening the weakness extends to lower extremities.

March 19. — Nervous trembling of hands. Pressure in frontal region, extending into root of nose, with a sensation as if a nail was being driven into the brain on the left side. Symptoms ameliorate towards evening.

March 20. — Before rising in the morning, sensation as of a foreign substance in the larynx; on rising, pain in the right hypochondrium, disappearing on pressure. Throat sore, growing worse in the afternoon. From four to eight, P.M., aching of right molar teeth, commencing in lower jaw and gradually extending to the upper of same side. After going to bed, colicky pains in umbilical region, with a desire to press them, but pressure aggravates; better on rising. Stomach feels empty. Pains shoot from right hypochondrium downwards.

March 21, ten, A.M. — Feeling as if the tongue had been cut in the middle, and was just healing up. Two, P.M. Aching of right molar teeth, lasting only a few minutes; returning at six, P.M., lasting the remainder of the evening. Seven, P.M. Sore throat; worse than yesterday. After going to bed, colic similar to that described yesterday, but not quite as severe.

March 22. — A dull, stupid feeling all day. Colic pains came on earlier than yesterday, and are of short duration.

March 23. — A feeling of dullness, and inability to pursue studies; otherwise well.

March 24. Took last of preparation last night. Three, P.M. Throbbing pains in the right hypochondrium.

March 25. — A general depression of spirits; no appetite.

March 26. — All the former symptoms, but greatly ameliorated.

March 27, six, P.M. — Itching of the right ear.

March 28. — Right ear inflamed, and somewhat swollen.

March 29. — Right ear broke out in white blisters on red base; copious discharge of a watery fluid on puncturing; shooting pains in ear, when lying on that side.

March 30. — Soreness and swelling of the lymphatic gland under right ear. Four, P.M. Steady, cutting pain in right hypochondrium.

March 31. — Vesicles on ear dried up, and cuticle desquamating. Aching in outer edge of ear, when lying down, relieved by pressure.

April 1. — No symptoms; perfectly well.

Second Proving.

April 8, 1867. — First dec. dil. taken same as in first proving. Seven, P.M. — Aching of right molar teeth, lower jaw.

April 9. — On rising in the morning, a feeling of pressure in frontal region, and in root of nose; dull, frontal headache all day.

April 10. — Soreness in the abdomen; occasional stitches in right hypochondrium; some colic after retiring at night.

April 11. — Colic pains in the morning before rising, with discharge of flatulence. Dull pains in the forehead; heavy feeling over the eyes; pressure in the nose. After going to bed at night, colic, with emission of flatulence and borborygmus; awakens from sleep.

Friday, April 12. — Before rising, colic, with excessively bitter taste in the mouth; headache all through cerebrum; relieved somewhat on rising; colic disappears on motion, but comes on at intervals all day, with frequent discharge of wind from the bowels. Occasional throbbing pain over eyes, first right, then left; nervous trembling of hands. Eruption under the right ear, discharging a watery fluid.

April 13. — Dull, heavy feeling in the head; severe pains in left iliac region, worse on motion, occasionally changing to right side. In the evening, when first lying down, intense throbbing pain, commencing in glans penis, and extending to left pubic region, and gradually disappearing. When lying on the back, a feeling of pressure on abdomen.

April 14. — Shooting pains in the head before rising in the morning. Nine, A.M. Throbbing pains in left hip, lasting only a few minutes. About noon, severe colic, which seems mostly on the right side. Nervousness; an unexpected noise startles and causes a shooting pain over the eyes. Dizziness when walking. Nervous twitching of upper lip, extending to left eye.

April 15.—Throbbing pains in gluteal region. Cramp-like pains in region of the heart. In the afternoon, a severe headache, with depression of spirits, and a feeling of anxiety about some unknown thing.

April 16.—Headache over the eyes; weakness of the whole body; the walls of the chest, especially, feel as if they would sink in. Disposition to worry about something, he hardly knows what. Throbbing pains over left temple, then over right; colic pains below umbilicus. After going to bed, severe throbbing pains over eyes, first right, then left. Took the last of the drug at night.

April 17.—Sensation of fullness in brain. When walking, a cramp-like pain in the sacral region, left side, so severe that he has to stand still until it passes off.

April 18.—Occasional pains in right hypochondrium, shooting downwards. Cutting pains over right eye, sometimes left.

April 19.—When bending the body, cramp-like pains in cardiac region. In the evening, walls of chest feel as if they had not power to expand when breathing.

April 20.—Sensation as if food was lodged between the teeth on right side, commencing on lower jaw, extending to upper; teeth feel as if elongated. Throbbing pain over right eye; intense itching on back of right hand. Eight, P. M. Throat sore on right side.

April 21.—Throbbing pain over right eye, sometimes shooting from the root of nose upward. Two, P.M. Throat sore on right side; passed off about four P.M. Seven, P.M. Some colic pains in the hypogastrium; toothache on right side.

April 22—Soreness and inflammation of fauces, worse on

right side; soft palate and uvula inflamed. Dorsum of tongue sore on right side, causing painful mastication and deglutition.

April 23.— Throat ulcerated on right side; right side of tongue inflamed, not swollen.

April 24. — Throat better. Throbbing pains in left temple.

April 27. — No symptoms, except a dull frontal headache.

April 28. — Severe throbbing headache on rising; weakness of the whole body; at times cold streaks run up and down the spine; great hoarseness of the voice; breath hot, eyes heavy; throbbing pains over left eye, also in right temporal region; throat sore; when coughing, head feels as if it would burst.

April 29. — Headache seems to be more in the cerebellum. In the afternoon, the nape of neck grows stiff, causing painful tension when moving.

April 30. — Sweat all last night. In the morning everything tastes and smells sour. Some throbbing pain in right temple. Swelling of lymphatic gland under right ear.

May 1, 1867. — Felt better generally; some pains in head on left side, but by evening the symptoms were all gone.

May 2. — In evening, intense itching of right ear.

May 3. — Ear swollen, little white vesicles rising under epidermis. Shooting and throbbing pains in right hypogastrium. A boil began to make its appearance on right side of forehead, (the first in his life).

May 4. — Swelling of ear increasing. Steady pain in left hypogastrium, continuing several hours.

May 5. — The white vesicles in ear assumed a purple tinge. Swelling of lymphatics was disappearing.

May 6. — Ear not so much swollen.

May 7. — Desquamation of cuticle of right ear; the blisters discharged water.

May 8. — A feeling of weakness through the whole body. Nausea, and bitter taste in the mouth; tongue coated yellow; headache; eyes heavy. Frequent eructations of wind from the stomach; a distressing feeling of emptiness in œsophagus. Aching of right molar teeth, lower jaw, after going to bed; also shooting pains from left ear down to the spine.

May 9, seven, A.M. — Stinging pains in right ear; great soreness of the ear during the day; the blisters on ear scab over, and become filled with a greenish-looking pus; moving jaws painful. Five, P.M. Pains in ear of intense throbbing nature, worse on moving and exposure to the air. When walking, wants to hold his hand over it; sometimes pains shoot from it to the boil on forehead.

May 10. — Dull, heavy feeling in frontal region; face swollen in front of right ear, and painful to the touch. The ear is not painful to-day; some pus is discharged, and the scabs desquamate. After retiring, aching of right molar teeth on lower jaw.

May 12. — A slight bruise on the large joint of little finger of right hand inflames and suppurates, causing painful tension of the fingers of that hand.

May 15. — Ear healing up; boil on forehead discharges some pus every day.

May 16. — Vesicular eruption on right hand, commencing at the sore on little finger and gradually extending upwards.

May 17. — The eruption appears under right ear, and gradually extends over the whole face and neck, and on right hip; burning and itching sensation in the eruptions; on scratching, they discharge water.

Saturday, 18. — Burning in eruptions, increased on exposure to air; much worse to-day than yesterday.

May 19. — No more burning or itching; the eruptions began to disappear, and by the 22d they were all gone, and desquamation of the cuticle had set in. The boil on forehead discharged no more, and by the 25th it had entirely disappeared. About the same time another one made its appearance on right side of the chin, which continued painful until

June 2d, when it discharged some purulent matter, and then began to pass off; by June 5th, it was all gone, and from that date he experienced no symptoms.

During the above proving, he kept an accurate account of the rate of pulse, and could not detect any change; once, April 28, the pulse ran as high as 90; but often, in apparent health, it has been higher than that; average, during proving, 72. Kept account of the specific quantity of urine, and found but little change; standard, 1019,—average during proving, 1023. Since the proving, one of the right molar teeth of lower jaw has commenced to decay, but whether the effect of the remedy, or not, was uncertain.

GENERALITIES.—Right side principally affected; symptoms more from right to left, from above downwards, and from within outwards. Aggravated towards evening and on lying down. Ameliorated on motion and on rising.

Note.—Dr. Bacmeister, his preceptor, thinks it will prove a valuable antipsoric remedy: he has prescribed it in a case of eruption similar to that described in this proving, and it worked like a charm, curing the case in a few days.

PROVINGS BY C. H. LUTES, M.D.

Prover of nervo-bilious temperament; age thirty years; of good health at the time. Proving made with mother tincture, taken in water.

FIRST PROVING.

February 22, 1867, two, P.M.—Took three drops. Half past three, P.M.—Three drops. Nine, P.M. (In bed); sharp, thin pain across abdomen from side to side, half an inch above umbilicus; comes in flashes, at intervals of about one minute; relieved by pressure. Awoke in after part of the night with heartburn, and a sensation of fine, violent agitation of all the muscles of the body and limbs, worse in hands and fingers. This sensation passed away gradually in about five minutes.

February 23, seven, A.M. — Six drops. Nine, A.M. Sensation of intoxication; fits of vertigo, lasting three to five minutes, relieved by moving about, but worse on sudden motion. Sensation as if all objects about him were in quick, violent agitation. Ten, A.M. Sensation of cold and numbness in hands; they feel clumsy and stiff, with tingling and prickling, as if recovering from cold. Eleven, A.M. Fits of vertigo not so frequent, but more decided; worse on sudden motion and bending forward. One, P.M. Vertigo only when stooping. Two, P.M. Vertigo all gone, but head feels a little muddled. Took six drops; no symptoms.

February 24, noon. — Seven drops. No symptoms. Half-past five, P.M. — Ten drops. Six, P.M. Dull, heavy, passive pain around the umbilicus, with a fine, active pain above umbilicus, across the abdomen; relieved by pressure. Seven, P.M. No symptoms after supper.

February 25, nine, A.M. — Ten drops. Eleven, A.M. Dull, constant, heavy pain in the umbilical region. Abdomen feels hollow, empty, caved in. Took ten drops. No symptoms.

Three, P.M. — Fifteen drops. No symptoms.

Second Proving.

April 15, 1867, nine, A.M. — Took five drops of the mother tincture. Ten, A.M. — Fifteen drops. Eleven, A M. Felt languid and lazy; had no inclination to stir; aversion to all muscular exertion; constant nausea, and feeling of uneasiness in umbilical region; abdomen felt caved in. Sensation of softness in abdomen, and as if its front walls were drawn in towards the spine; dull, heavy pain in umbilical region. Abdomen weak, lax; sick; wanted to be let alone. Pulsations in umbilicus isochronous with those of the heart. One, P.M. Symptoms gone.

Three, P.M. — Took ten drops. At half past four, P.M. — Fifteen drops. Five, P.M. Dull, heavy, aching in region of umbilicus; abdomen feels caved in, with sense of heat; general feeling of muscular weakness; inclination to avoid all exertion, mental and muscular; sensation as if the nervous system were resting; flushes of heat in abdomen. Half past five, P.M. Prickling numbness in hands; sensation as if they were cold, and larger than usual. Six, P.M. Feeling in hands like that produced by electricity. Symptoms in the abdomen nearly gone. Nine, P.M. Beating in abdomen; tingling in hands and fingers; head feels light; mind confused; intolerance of loud talking. A voice usually pleasant sounds very coarse and rough; thought that it would produce spasms if he were obliged to listen. Impression produced by the sound heard last continues a long time.

April 16, half past five, A.M. — Ten drops. Ten, A.M. — Fifteen drops. No symptoms.

April 17, nine, A.M. — Twenty drops. Noon. — Twenty drops. In half an hour, a feeling of warmth in abdomen and stomach; dull pain in abdomen; general feeling of intoxication. Brain seems agitated, mind confused, pupils contracted; sensation as if all objects were in violent agitation; nothing seems to be at rest. One, P.M. Symptoms all less marked. Three, P.M. — Symptoms gone. Took twenty drops; no symptoms.

Proving discontinued for want of time to attend to it.

Remark. — The above proving, though not very satisfactory to the prover, was not spun out, and made up from imagination. No symptoms were given but those well marked, and which could not reasonably be attributed to any cause but that of the drug. C. H. L.

PROVINGS BY C. W. PIERCE, M.D.

Prover in good health, but having from birth a tendency to unnatural desquamation of the skin.

First Proving.

Nov. 12, 1867, nine, P.M. — Took ten drops, mother tincture, in one ounce of water. Slept well until two, A.M., when he awoke, dreaming of fighting.

Nov. 13, seven, A.M. — Ten drops. Nine, A.M. A sharp, darting pain through upper lobe of left lung, lasting only a short time, but returning every half-hour; aggravated by descending stairs; did not feel it after the first day.

Noon. — Ten drops. Appetite very good. A feeling of mental uneasiness, wandering from one subject to another.

Nine, P.M. — Ten drops. Was quite hungry, but did not eat very heartily. Had most frightful dreams; dreamed of getting whipped, and killing snakes.

Nov. 14, seven, A.M. — Twenty drops. Had an abnormal appetite, but his food did not distress him. After eating, a feeling of liveliness and activity for one hour; next hour, gradual passing off of cheerfulness, amounting to sadness, and a disposition to be displeased with everybody and everything. Could not concentrate his thoughts. Soreness and weariness in lower extremities.

Noon. — Took twenty drops. One, P.M. Felt a sharp, darting pain through left superciliary ridge, extending deep into the head, lasting but a short time; would return at intervals, whether in motion or not. A prickling in lower extremities, almost like that of pins, mostly in popliteal space; on scratching, it burns like fire, but no change in color of the skin.

Nine, P.M. — Twenty drops. Dreamed as before. Had a dull, heavy headache in frontal region; burning in the skin of lower extremities like fire. Could get more relief from rubbing than scratching.

Nov. 15, seven, A.M. — Sixty drops. Feeling, as before, of liveliness after eating, followed by great depression of spirits. Red spots on lower extremities, alike in position on both; after an hour or so, they would change to a purple color; there would be no itching quite near or on the spots, but around on the healthy skin. Weakness and depression all over the body, especially in lower extremities.

Noon. — Took sixty drops. Felt all the afternoon as though he would break out into a profuse perspiration, but did not. Bright-red spots in various parts of the body, changing as before to a purple color.

Ten, P.M. — Sixty drops. Could go to sleep quite easily; was able to sleep only a short time, awaking from horrible dreams, and covered with a profuse perspiration. Itching was not so annoying while perspiring.

Nov. 16, seven, A.M. — One hundred drops. One hour before breakfast counted as many as fifty spots on various parts of the body, most of them on upper and lower extremities; one or two on the chest. Itching more confined to the trunk. Discontinued the use of the drug for two weeks, during which time the itching continued as annoying as ever. By getting in the least degree excited or warmed, the spots would be as red as ever, but in an hour or so would subside and assume a purple hue. After the expiration of two weeks, could see where the spots had been. The itching was as annoying as ever; it did not produce any disorganization of the skin. As the spots disappeared, they became of a dirty-yellow color, somewhat like that left by a bruise. Appetite remained quite good for two weeks.

Second Proving.

Nov. 30, 1867. — Took ten drops of the first dec. dil. three times a day for three days. Did not get any prominent symptoms, and discontinued the use of the drug.

PROVING BY MRS. W.

Reported by Dr. Pierce.

Prover aged thirty-five; of a bilious temperament; took the drug for three days.

Nov. 12–14, inclusive.—Three times per day. The first day, ten drops at a time; second day, twenty; third, sixty. It occasioned quite an irritation of the skin, but not the peculiar spots manifested in the preceding case. The itching was so intense all over the body that she could not be induced to continue the proving longer. She described it as so many thousand fleas on her; could not refrain from constant scratching. The itching was not worse at night. The drug did not seem to have any other effect upon her.

PROVINGS BY A. V. MARSHALL, M.D.

First Proving.

To one hundred grains of sugar-of-milk, on which Prof. Hale had dropped one hundred drops of the tincture, the prover added one and a half ounces of alcohol. Of this solution he took a dose four times a day, commencing with three drops and gradually increasing, till, at last, he took drachm doses, until the preparation was all gone. No symptoms could be found.

Second Proving.

He then waited four days and commenced taking the first decimal trituration, in three-grain doses, four times a day, gradually increasing the dose to fifteen grains, when fifty grains (all which Dr. Hale had sent) were exhausted. During the last three or four days, there was a peculiar reddish-clouded appearance of the skin over the whole body. Aside from that, he remained perfectly healthy, taking his usual meals without tea or coffee.

Bowels continued to move once a day, as usual; would not have known from his feelings that he had taken any drug. Two days after discontinuing the drug, the clouded appearance of the skin disappeared.

Third Proving.

April 13, 1867. — Took one scruple of Ptelein, one-fifth, at three different times on an empty stomach, and continued to take it in the same manner for four succeeding days. Felt as well as usual till evening, when suddenly had a severe urging to stool; it was very loose and dark-colored. The diarrhœa did not continue.

April 14. — Bowels regular.

April 15. — No symptoms.

April 16. — Rose with a dull headache, which wore away after an hour or two. Had dreamed of armies of soldiers rising out of their graves, and marching into the house. Bowels regular. Occasional pains in various parts of the abdomen throughout the day. Went to bed at half past eight, P.M. Dropped to sleep, and at nine o'clock was awakened by a painful urging to stool; it proved to be another attack of diarrhœa; quantity small, but with much pain throughout the bowels.

April 17. — Dull headache in morning. Had dreamed of enemies prowling about the house. Felt a soreness about the abdomen, aggravated more by bending the body in any direction than by pressure. The soreness or heaviness of the bowels is such as to incline him, when sitting or walking, to support the abdomen with the hands, indicating a moderate degree of congestion of the abdominal viscera. Appetite about the same as usual, except that he gets tired before he gets through eating. Yesterday the tongue was slightly swollen, and had white fur on it; more of swelling and fur to-day, with burning of the mouth and lips as if touched with tincture of Aconite. After taking the drug, had sour stomach and a dull, heavy pain, extending around the small of the back.

April 18. — Rose with a headache; brassy taste in mouth; stomach sour; bowels costive. and not so sore as yesterday. The soreness or lameness of the lumbar region is worse. Same doses. Pain in the lower part of each lung in the evening.

April 19. — Rose with a headache and general soreness of the body, and wandering pains about the limbs. Pain in lumbar region most of the time, and sometimes in the right hip.

April 22. — Symptoms similar to those on the 19th, except there is less energy and less appetite.

April 25. — The symptoms have gradually worn away.

May 1, 1867. — For some days has felt free from the influence of the drug. Has no acquaintance with it, except from these provings. Would think it might be of use in treating certain rheumatic cases in aged people, in which there is a general soreness of the body and limbs; and especially of the abdominal and lumbar regions, with alternate diarrhœa and constipation. Possibly it may be of use in some forms of skin disease.

PROVING BY E. PARSONS, M.D.

Jan. 12, 1867, ten, A.M.—Commenced the proving by taking fifty drops of the tincture. Noon. — Took fifty drops. After this, experienced slight nausea and giddiness. Sharp, darting pains through the forehead and temples.

Half past two, P.M. — Fifty drops. Half past three. Confusion of ideas, and drowsiness.

Half past four, P.M. — Fifty drops.

Jan. 13, nine, A.M. — Fifty drops. Ten, A.M. A severe pain in the region of the heart, lasting several minutes. Eleven, A.M. Severe pain in the left leg, three inches below the knee. Half an hour after, severe darting pain in the right temple, and throbbing pains in the left supra-orbital region. Fifty drops at half past one, half past five, and at nine, P.M. Retired about half past ten. Severe, sharp, darting pains in the right thigh;

pains seemed to be muscular, and lasting for several minutes; also severe darting pains through forehead.

Jan. 14. — Before rising, felt pricking pains through and in the throat, particularly in the tonsils and larynx, lasting several minutes, and quite severe; roaring in the ears. Half past eight. — Fifty drops. Extreme lassitude; disinclination for mental labor or bodily exertion. Heaviness of the head, with a muddled feeling, and dull, aching pain in forehead. Took fifty drops at ten, A.M., at noon, and at two, P.M. Giddiness, dullness, and languor.

Four, P.M. — Fifty drops. Soon after this experienced severe darting and throbbing pains in the left supra-orbital region.

Eight, P.M. — Fifty drops, soon followed by a sensation as if diarrhœa would come on. Sleep heavy, and troubled with dreams of robbers, &c.

Jan. 15. — Took fifty drops at nine, A.M., noon, and three, P.M. Extreme lassitude. Pain in left lung, lasting for several minutes. Roaring in the ears. Disinclination for mental labor. Severe darting pains just above the supra-orbital ridge.

Six, P.M. — Fifty drops. Severe darting pains in right temporal region. Half past nine. — Fifty drops. Pain in carious tooth, with extreme sensitiveness; soreness of the gums. All the teeth feel sensitive, with a dull, aching pain. Pulse 85, regular, full; normal pulse 75. Ten, P.M. Pain and rumbling in bowels, as if diarrhœa would supervene. Severe frontal headache. The pain throbbing. Half past ten. Pain and rumbling in bowels, with copious evacuation. Chilliness, with great sensitiveness to cold air, and desire to be near the fire. General feeling of *malaise*, with aching in the lower extremities, and premonitory symptoms of fever.

Jan. 16. — Took fifty drops at nine, A.M., noon, three and seven, P.M. Felt very badly all day. Dull, aching pain through forehead and temples; roaring in the ears; severe pain in the lower extremities, worse on standing. Weakness, with disinclination to move or study; chilliness, and extreme sensitiveness to cold air. Pulse 85. Urine scanty, with copious deposit of phosphates and epithelial scales. Sp. gr. 1035.

Jan. 17. — Fifty drops at nine, A.M., noon, three, five, and seven, P.M. — Felt better this morning, but in the afternoon felt quite badly again, with pain in the forehead and temples, aching in the limbs, dullness, drowsiness, and incontinence of urine. Sp. gr. 1035. A free deposit of phosphates. Constipation. Pulse 80.

Jan. 18. — Fifty drops at half past eight and eleven, A.M., two and six, P.M. Felt better in the morning, but in the afternoon and evening much worse again. Pains to day worse in the right side. Pains in the right leg, below the knee, extending to the ankle. Dull, aching pain in the small of the back. Pain in right zygoma, and in the right temple; also in the forehead. Nose stuffed up; sneezing; soreness of nasal passages; influenza. Pulse 80. Urine frequent, rather scanty, some scalding, and difficulty of retention. Sp. gr. 1030. Deposit less copious.

Jan. 19. — Fifty drops at nine, A.M., noon, and four, P.M. Felt much better to-day till half past four, when the pains of the extremities, back, and head all returned. Pains in head quite severe at half past nine, P.M. Pulse 84. Urine scanty during the day; the scalding and difficulty of retention all gone. Sp. gr. 1030.

Jan. 20. — Took no medicine. Feel some better. Catarrhal symptoms still continue, but less violent. Pain in the head, limbs, etc., not so severe. Urine slightly alkaline; copious deposit of phosphates and urates, tinged with purpurine. Sp. gr. 1035.

Jan. 21. — Awoke about two, A.M., with severe pains in forehead, roaring in the ears, and very severe pain in right kidney. Very restless and uneasy, rolling and tossing about. Could not get to sleep for a long time, from pain and restlessness. In the morning felt some better. Pain in kidney relieved. Slight pain in the head, and roaring in the ears, which increase in severity towards evening. In the evening, while riding on cars, had a severe pain in right forearm, lasting several minutes. The pain seemed to be in the flexor muscles of the forearm.

This ended the proving; all the unpleasant symptoms gradually disappeared, and at the end of a week he felt as well as usual.

Remark. — The prover was naturally of a costive habit, and was costive when he commenced the proving. But, after taking the drug, the bowels moved regularly every morning, without any particular uneasiness, for two or three days, when symptoms of diarrhœa came on, which, however, amounted only to one thorough operation as from cathartic action. After this the bowels became constipated again, there being no movement for two or three days at a time.

The appetite was much increased for the first few days of the proving, after which it diminished. No particular loathing of food, but rather an indifference to it.

The sexual appetite was very much increased for several days, after which there was a total absence of sexual excitement, until the medicine was discontinued.

PROVING BY A. HAYWARD, M.D.

Prover, aged thirty-seven, nervo-bilious temperament, health good.

April 17, 1867, eleven, A.M. — Took two grains of the third decimal trituration, and again at three, P.M.

April 18.— Sleep natural. No symptoms. Took doses of two grains, at six and ten, A.M. Frontal headache. Two, P.M. —Two grains. Dull headache throughout the head. Six, P.M. —Two grains. Severe pains in forehead and occiput.

April 19.—Slept well. Very little pain in the morning. Four grains at nine, A.M., and again at two, P.M. Head nearly free from pain. Nine, P.M.— Four grains. Not much headache.

April 20. — Very little headache; sleep natural. Doses of six grains at six, ten, two, and six, P.M. Symptoms unchanged.

April 21. — No symptoms. Doses of ten grains at eight, A.M., noon, and four, P.M.

April 22. — Doses of fifteen grains at eight, A.M., noon, four, and nine, P.M. No symptoms.

April 23. — Doses of fifteen grains at six and nine, A.M. No symptoms. Two, P.M.—Frontal headache. Fifteen grains; and again at five, P.M.; slight ptyalism and headache.

April 24, six, A.M. — Slight ptyalism and headache. Twenty grains; again at ten, and at three, P.M. Ptyalism, but head nearly free from pain. Slight burning in throat and stomach.

April 25. — Doses of twenty grains at eight, eleven, A.M., three, six, and nine, P.M. No symptoms during the day, except slight ptyalism and a little dull headache.

April 26. — Doses of twenty grains at six and ten, A.M., and three, P.M. Headache and slight sickness at stomach.

April 27 to 30. — Took doses of twenty grains four times a day, about three hours apart. No symptoms, except slight headache and ptyalism. Tongue smarts and prickles, and burns a little.

May 1 to 4. — Took daily four doses of twenty grains, three hours apart. No symptoms

May 5 to 11. — Took daily three doses of twenty grains four hours apart. No symptoms.

May 12. — Two doses of two grains, first dec. trit., six hours apart. No symptoms.

May 13. — Doses of two grains at six and nine, A.M., three and six, P.M. Slight salivation. Out of medicine.

PROVING BY G. C. HUNTER, M.D.

Prover 45 years of age; temperament bilious, nervous, and lymphatic, — bilious predominating; weight one hundred and ninety-five pounds; slightly dyspeptic.

April 19, 1867. — Took five doses of thirty drops each of the saturated tincture of the fresh root, commencing at half past ten, A.M.

April 21. — Took six doses of thirty drops each.

April 22, eleven, A.M. — Took eighty drops, which was all he had prepared. He took in all four hundred and ten drops. Could not say that he felt the slightest unusual symptom during the time or since. Concluded that either his tincture was worthless, or that he was not a good subject for proving it.

CLINICAL OBSERVATIONS ON PTELEA.

PTYRIASIS VERSICOLOR. A middle-aged man was covered with this eruption on all parts of the body except hands and face. He had all the usual characteristics of the disease. He had tried Arsenicum, Kali iod. and Sarsaparilla, with no good results. Ptelea, second dil., ten drops three times daily, cured the case in six weeks.

E. M. HALE.

CHRONIC GASTRITIS.—A middle-aged woman had for several years a constant sensation of corrosion, heat, or burning in the stomach; occasional vomiting of ingesta, constipation; fever every afternoon; lowness of spirits, and debility. She had taken Nux vom., Carbo veg., Phosphorus, and several other remedies, with only temporary benefit. Ptelea, second dil., ten drops in a spoonful of water before each meal, effected a permanent cure in five weeks.

P. H. HALE.

ERYSIPELAS. —Two cases of erysipelas came under my treatment, in which quinia and iron had been used in large doses without succcss, and rather with injury to the patient. A rapid recovery ensued after the use of Ptelea.

DR. MILLER.

ICTERUS, WITH HYPERÆMIA OF THE LIVER.—In severe cases of this disease, I have found Ptelea an excellent remedy. Ptelea primarily affects the liver; the stools are generally of a brown or gray color, with considerable odor.

DR. MILLER.

Asthma.—In two cases of asthma, Ptelea was of more service than any other remedy. DR. MILLER.

Ascites.—I found Ptelea to cure a case of ascites of very severe type after many agents had been employed without success. DR. MILLER.

Phthisis.—Several cases of hectic fever, with purulent expectoration of a sweetish taste, but without any other chest symptom than a slight mucous rhonchus, and sibilant râle, were cured completely with Ptelea. DR. MILLER.

RESUME OF PTELEA TRIFOLIATA.

[*Explanation of Symbols.* — (·) A pathogenetic symptom not confirmed by clinical experience. (*) Confirmed by clinical experience. (o) Curative, but not observed as pathogenetic. (v) Verified by one or more other provers. The symptoms in *Italics* denote the *persistence* of a symptom in all the provings. *With* in Italics couples symptoms of two classes.]

Mind and Disposition.

1 · *Great languor* and *indisposition* for either mental or physical labor (vvvv).

· Malaise of body and mind (vv); desire to lie down and think of nothing at all.

· Inability to concentrate the thoughts; they seem chasing each other through the brain.

· Complete incapacity for mental exertion, with headache (vv).

5 · Fretful and irritable at very slight causes (vv).

·· Compelled to give up any attempt at exertion in P.M.

· *Performed his duties in a perfunctory manner.*

· *Great mental confusion* (vv).

· The mind moves slowly and heavily; with difficulty in remembering familiar things.

10 ·Extraordinary weakness of memory; inability to recall familiar names.

·Peevish, irritable feeling, and intolerance of noise (v).

·*Marked forgetfulness*, with increased headache, and disposition to hurry when writing.

·Great forgetfulness, and yet an ability, on collecting the thoughts, to recall things read many years ago.

·Confusion of thought, with hurriedness of manner; forgetfulness, with mistakes in writing. (From a large dose.)

15 ·Sick and faint (v); desire to shrink from any mental work.

·Dull and stupid feeling (v).

·Great depression of spirits, *with* sour stomach.

·Aversion to society; a wish to be let alone (v).

·Annoyance and irritation from ordinary conversation (v).

20 ·Liveliness for an hour after eating, followed by great depression and sadness.

Head.

·Pressive feeling at the base of the brain, with nausea, closely resembling the Ipecac symptom; "Headache as if the brain and skull were bruised, penetrating through all the bones down to the root of the tongue, with nausea."

·Frontal headache all day (vvvv); pressing from within outwards.

·Pressive pain in the frontal region, extending to the roots of the nose, as if a nail were driven into the brain (left side).

·Piercing pain shooting through the temples (vv), *with* increased headache and nausea.

25 ·Splitting headache, *with* nausea.

·Piercing pain in the brain, *with* giddiness, and severe aching pain in the stomach.

·Headache after dinner, aggravated by mental exertion.

· Sharp, cutting pains through the front of the brain, alleviated by pressure.

· *Racking frontal headache,* with heat of the face and head, and great desire to hurry his business.

30 · Heaviness in the occiput, with a gloomy feeling in the forehead.

· Heavy, pressive frontal headache, worse at night, pressing from within outwards, and aggravated by stooping.

· Stunning, pressing headache (a similar one was cured by Rhus).

· Head feels languid and heavy, with inability to follow a connected train of thought.

· Persistent headache, with sharp pains shooting from the frontal to the left parietal region.

35 · Frontal headache, aggravated by moving the eyes, and by noise.

· Frontal headache deep in the brain.

· Sudden, pressive pains in the temples, worse in the right (vvv).

· Fine, neuralgic pains in the temples, worse in the right.

· *Constant dull headache* (vv), aggravated by going upstairs, and by walking.

40 · Sharp, darting pain over the left eye, extending deep into the brain.

· Throbbing pains over the eyes, from right to left.

· Shooting pains in the head, before rising in the morning (vv).

· Throbbing pains over the temples, from left to right.

· Severe throbbing headache on rising, with great weakness.

45 · Dull, frontal headache, with depression and sour stomach.

· Headache intermitting with pain in the hypogastrium, dizziness, and nausea.

· Pain in the left side of the head and right side of the neck.

· Headache over the eyes (v).

· Sudden pressive pain in the temples, as if they would be pressed together, or as if the right would be pressed to the left (frequently recurring during the proving).

50 · Frontal and occipital headache (vvv).

· Headache while reading (v).

Sensorium.

· Giddiness on rising in the morning.

· Giddiness, with continual vertigo and increased abdominal tenderness.

· Giddiness of the head, and, when walking, reeling as if intoxicated (vv).

55 · Giddiness and vertigo in A.M., so as to necessitate a recumbent posture.

· Severe attack of vertigo, with increased headache, and aggravation of all the symptoms.

· Sudden giddiness, with faintness on turning the head; vertigo aggravated by even a gradual turning of the head.

· Vertigo and nausea, aggravated by rising to the feet, also by walking; inability to stand without the aid of a chair.

· Vertigo and confusion too severe to permit letter-writing.

60 · Sudden atttack of vertigo, lasting a minute.

· Everything seemed to be in violent agitation.

Eyes.

· Twitching of the eyelids.

· A shooting pain over the eyes when startled.

· Nervous twitching of the upper lip, extending to left eye.

65 ·Nervous pain, extending from the left arm to left eye.

·Rolling the eyes upwards aggravated the frontal headache.

·Pressure over the eyes, aggravated by lifting the eyebrows.

·Heavy feeling over the eyes (v).

·Pain in the eyes (v).

70 ·Pupils contracted.

·Painful sensitiveness to light, with irritability.

Ears.

·Ringing in the ears, with slight giddiness.

·Sensitiveness to sounds (v); impression of sounds last heard continues for a long time.

·Intolerance of noise, and of loud talking; annoyance at even ordinary conversation.

75 ·Easily startled at unusual sounds.

·Pain in the right ear.

·Continuous pain behind the right ear.

·Intense throbbing pain in the ear, worse on motion.

·Itching of the right ear, with inflammation and swelling, terminating in white blisters on a red base, discharging a copious, watery fluid. (Occurred twice on the same spot.)

Face, etc.

80 ·Burning heat of cheeks and face (v).

·Heat of head and face, especially of the forehead.

·Yellowish face, with dry, hot skin (v).

·Sickly paleness of the face, especially around the eyes.

·Pressure at the roots of the nose (v).

Mouth, Tongue, etc.

85 ·Feverishness and dryness of the lips, with thirst. (Primary.)

· The lips cracked and sore, notwithstanding an abundance of saliva. (Secondary.)

· Burning, prickling sensation of the mouth and tongue.

· Much dryness of the lips and tongue, *with* hawking of mucous from the pharynx.

· Great dryness of the mouth, with bitter taste.

90 · Great dryness of the mouth and throat (v).

· Increased secretion of saliva of a saltish or bitter taste.

· Drooling in the night, wetting the pillow.

· Fine prickling sensation over the whole surface of the tongue (vvv).

· Tongue coated with a yellowish fur; the papillæ red and prominent.

95 · Tongue dry and brownish-yellow, or light-brown (v).

· Tongue swollen (v), and furred; white.

· Tongue coated yellow along the centre and base (v).

· Tongue feeling as if it had been cut through the middle and was now healing up.

· Tongue feeling as if scalded, or as after taking Aconite.

100 · Tongue inflamed (vvv), but not swollen.

Jaws and Teeth.

· Dull, aching pains in all the teeth.

· Teeth all feel sore, *with* increased secretion of saltish saliva.

· Pain in the right molar teeth; first lower, then upper.

· Teeth feeling elongated, and as if something was crowding them apart.

105 · Pain when moving the jaws.

Throat.

· Roughness of the fauces, with nausea (v).

· Sensation as of a foreign body in the larynx.

· Slight vertigo, *with* a choking feeling in the pharnyx (at evening).

· Soreness and inflammation of the fauces (vvv), soft palate, and uvula (worse on right side).

110 · Throat ulcerated and tongue inflamed (right side).

· Distressing feeling of emptiness in the œsophagus.

· Slight burning in the throat and stomach.

· Hiccough.

· Sense of obstruction in the larynx on waking.

115 · Great hoarseness; inability to speak aloud (vv).

Taste and Appetite.

· Appetite increased (vvvvv). (Primary.)

· Unusual hunger; craving for acid food.

· Voracious appetite; food had not its natural taste; *with* pain in epigastrium following every meal; despondency.

· Appetite poor (vvvv); but little appetite and no thirst.

120 · Bread seemed tasteless; all other food tasteless or unnatural.

· Great repugnance to animal food; and to rich puddings, of which he is ordinarily fond.

· *Grea repugnance to butter* and fatty foods; even a small quantity aggravated the epigastric pain.

· Disgust at the sight or smell of food, especially of roast beef.

· The taste of the medicine continually returning in gusts to the mouth, with a feeling as if vomiting would relieve.

125 · Very little appetite (vv), with great repugnance to butter.

· Eructations tasting of the medicine, with persistent nausea (v).

· Eructations tasting of rotten eggs.

· Sour eructations (vvv).

·Frequent bitter taste in the mouth (vv), with dryness.

130 ·Taste of brass on rising in the morning.

Gastric Derangements.

·Slight but persistent nausea (vvv).

·Nausea and retching, *with* increase of frontal headache; aggravated by speaking.

·Severe nausea, with efforts to vomit, for two minutes.

135 ·Sensation of goneness, or an empty feeling in the stomach after eating.

·Nausea, with distress in the umbilical region, and headache (vv).

·Increased nausea, with heat of skin and profuse perspiration on the forehead (vv), after dinner.

·Sensation of repletion and fullness after a meal.

·Nausea and vomiting, without relief from the frontal headache (vv).

140 · *Persistent nausea* (vvvv) and vomiting, *with* giddiness and unsteadiness of the legs; aggravated by walking (v).

·Awakened at one, A.M., by a pressing pain in the stomach, as of a weight; aggravated by motion and pressure, accompanied with eructations of a bitter fluid, with deathly nausea, confusion of head, and sweat on the forehead. (The attack lasted four hours, and resembled acute dyspepsia.)

·Eructations, which almost caused emesis (after stool).

·Griping in the epigastric region, *with* dryness of the mouth, yellow-coated tongue, and a bitter taste (v).

·Eructations of bitter fluid, with deathly nausea.

145 ·Colic, with emission of flatus, and borborygmus (vv).

·Emission of flatus, relieved by motion.

Remark. — All the gastric symptoms were much aggravated after meals.

HEPATIC SYMPTOMS.

· Sharp pains in the right hypochondrium (vv).

· Constant feeling of weight in both hypochondria when walking; a dragging pain (vv).

· Sharp, cutting pain in right hypochondrium, aggravated by a deep inspiration (while in bed).

150 · Occasional pains in right hypochondrium, shooting downwards (v).

· Dull, heavy pain, apparently on the convex surface of the liver.

· Liver perceptibly swollen and sore on pressure, causing a dull, aching pain, with stitches.

· Awakened by a dull, heavy pain in the liver, relieved by lying on the right side. A feeling, when lying on the left side, as of the liver dragging on its ligaments.

· Liver swollen, and tender to a light touch.

155 · Heavy, aching pain in the liver, *with* deficient appetite.

· Sharp pains in the right hypochondriac and epigastric regions, caused by rapid motion.

· Awoke with hard, aching distress in the base of the liver (v).

· Hepatic and gastric symptoms, aggravated towards morning, awaking the prover at four o'clock.

° Tertian ague, with profuse vomiting of bilious matters.

160 ° Attacks of quartan ague, continuing for two years, resisting many remedies.

STOMACH AND ABDOMEN.

· Tenderness of the splenic region, with soreness on pressure (vv).

· Abdomen swollen and tender, with severe splenic pain (vv).

· Severe abdominal pain near umbilicus (vvv). Worse on motion.

· Sharp stitch proceeding from the umbilicus towards the spine when taking a deep inspiration, with increased tenderness on pressure.

165 · A faint feeling in the stomach, with sourish eructations (v).

· A squeezing pain in the epigastrium, worse in bed, with swollen but not painful abdomen.

· Aching of the bowels while walking (v).

· Throbbing, griping pains in the epigastrium, aggravated by a full, deep inspiration, by speaking, and by pressure, causing nausea.

· Pain and soreness across the abdomen, and in the epigastrium (vvv), aggravated by standing or sitting erect, and relieved by stooping forwards.

170 · Rumbling in the umbilical region, and swelling, with slight vertigo, and sweat on the forehead.

· *Rumbling in the bowels* (vvvv), and bloating, *with* tenderness on pressure.

· Burning and qualmishness at the stomach, *with* pain on pressure.

· Griping, contractive pain in the stomach, moving downwards (v).

· Griping, worse on pressure, in the bowels, *with* rumbling and bloating.

175 · Pressure as of a stone at the pit of the stomach (vv), aggravated by a light meal.

· Colicky pains in the small intestines (during the evening).

· Flying pains in the abdomen, with desire for stool.

· Stomach feels empty after eating; a sensation of "goneness" (v).

· Severe aching distress in the left hypochondrium (vv).

180 ·Frequent drawing pains in the epigastric and umbilical regions (vvv).

·Stitches in the abdomen, relieved by pressure (v).

·Pain in the epigastrium, *with* nausea (vv).

·Severe pains in the left iliac region, changing to the right; worse on motion.

·Severe, bearing-down pains in the bowels; spasmodic and griping, or sharp and throbbing.

185 ·*Pain in the hypogastrium* (vv) and bladder, *with* headache, intermitting during the paroxyms.

·*Retraction of the abdomen* (vvv), *with* pulsations isochronous with the heart.

·Soreness of the abdomen, aggravated by motion, and relieved by carrying it with the hands (vv).

·Abdomen tender on pressure for three weeks after the proving.

STOOL AND ANUS.

·Sudden and unexpected urging to go to stool, which was diarrhœic, with slight tenesmus, accompanied by sweat on the forehead and head (vv).

190 ·Urging before stool, *with* straining during a diarrhœic stool.

·*Constipation* (vvvv), with a continual urging in the rectum.

·Constant urging to stool, with rumbling in the bowels all day (vvv).

·*Small, hard stool,* with much straining (vvv).

·Hard and difficult stool, followed by smarting of the anus (vv).

195 ·Stools of usual consistence, with slimy coating, accompanied with straining and vertigo.

·Involuntary discharge of flatus, with ineffectual urging to stool.

· Urging to stool, with difficult passage of balls of hardened fæces.

· *Constant ineffectual urging to stool; a continual pressure in the rectum* (vv).

· Pressure in the rectum all day, resulting in the discharge of a small stool of indurated fæces, with slight relief; apparently a true torpor of the rectum.

200 · Pressure in the rectum, with qualmishness, aggravated by motion. (From a dose of five hundred drops. See, also, the next five symptoms).

· Violent urging, followed by a stool of fluid consistence and fetid smell; the passage accompanied with chilliness and shivering; and, after this, renewed tenesmus.

· Urging to stool, and sudden copious discharge of thin diarrhœic fæces, of a cadaverous smell, *with* smarting of the anus.

· Pressure in the rectum, as in dysentery, not relieved by a stool.

· Two stools in succession of fæces coated with mucus, followed by *tenesmus;* during stool, shuddering and chilliness of sacral region; after stool, smarting of the anus, with itching.

205 · Copious stool of fluid consistence and bilious smell; with it was a very copious expulsion of ascarides.

· Diarrhœic stools of a dark color, and sulphurous smell.

· Distress in the small intestines before stool.

· Mushy stools.

· Dark-colored, lumpy stools.

Sexual Organs, — Male.

210 · Intense throbbing pain in the glans penis, extending into the pubic region, when retiring.

· Increase of sexual desire at night.

· Lascivious dreams in the morning.

Sexual Organs, — Female.

· Catamenia two days too early, and quite copious (after continued exertion).

Urinary Organs.

· *High-colored urine* (vv).

215 · Urine of a deep color, and scalding slightly during its passage (v).

· Urine high-colored; the yellowish-red of Neubauer and Vogel.

· Urine redder than usual during the whole proving (v).

· Urine scanty, and of a deep-reddish or reddish-yellow tint, during the whole proving.

· Urine less, with a reddish, cloudy sediment.

220 · Urine profuse, and of a light color; the quantity decreased and then increased during the proving.

· A deposit of muddy sediment in the urine; afterwards whitish, with increase in quantity.

· Pain in the region of the bladder, with headache intermitting.

· Pain in the stomach and bladder.

· Uneasiness in the bladder and prostate gland; obliged to rise in the night to urinate.

225 · Pain in the prostatic region.

· Tickling and uneasiness in the urethra after urinating.

· Smarting sensation in the urethra while urinating.

· Burning in the urethra.

Remark. — The quantity of urine increased each day, and afterwards slightly decreased (during two provings). The condition of the kidneys improved by the proving.

Respiratory Organs.

· Aching pain, *with* occasional stitches, in the region of the diaphragm.

230 · Stitches in the diaphragm, arising from continued speaking.

· Stitching pains in the upper part of the posterior mediastinum, aggravated by breathing or a recumbent position, and accompanied with soreness of the trapezius muscles.

· Pressure on the lungs, with a sense of suffocation.

· Uneasiness and difficulty of breathing, coming on as the gastric and hepatic symptoms declined; with dull pain especially in the right infra-clavicular region, accompanied by —

· Hacking cough, without expectoration. This has approached very insidiously, and now —

235 · The right lung is dull on percussion at the apex.

· During a full inspiration, sharp pains shoot from the sternum towards the nipples; worse on the left.

· Pressure on the intercostal spaces, close to the sternum, causes a dull, aching pain.

Remark. — These thoracic symptoms are better in the house, and aggravated in the keen air. (Secondary.) By T. N. from the tincture.]

· Cough, with bursting headache, in the morning.

· A sharp, darting pain through the upper part of left lung; frequently returning, and aggravated by stepping downwards.

240 · Pain in the lower part of each lung, in the evening.

· Stitches through the right lung, which is sound.

· Pain back of the left breast, near the axilla.

· Pain under the right breast.

· Cramp-like pain in the cardiac region (v).

245 · Dyspnœa; the walls of the chest feel as though they would sink in (vv).

Back and Neck.

· Severe aching in the lumbar and sacral regions (vvvv).

· Dull backache every morning on waking (vv).

· Hard, aching distress in the dorsal region, for an hour in the morning (vv).

· Pains in the left scapula, aggravated by the exertion of writing.

250 · Bruised sensation in all the limbs and back; worse on pressure.

· Rending, tearing pains in the left scapula.

· Drawing, aching pains in the left scapula and shoulder-joint (vv).

· Dull, aching pain in the small of the back, aggravated by motion.

· Severe pains in the back, worse in dorsal region, disturbing sleep.

255 · Awakened by aggravated pains in the lumbar region.

· Hard backache the whole length of spine and back of the neck, also through the right shoulder.

· Walking arrested by a cramp-like pain in the left sacral region.

· Lameness in the cords of the neck, right side.

· The whole neck feels swollen.

260 · Dull, heavy pain and soreness in the lumbar region.

Upper Extremities.

· A tingling, prickling in the hands and fingers, like that produced by electricity (vv).

· A prickling numbness in the hands, which seem larger than usual and clumsy (vv).

· Fine, sharp pains in the fingers.

· Dull, aching distress in the hands and fingers.

265 · Hands and feet are hot, dry, and feverish (vv).

· Hands and fingers cold, numb, clumsy, and stiff (vv).

· Dull pains in the elbows and wrists.

· Frequent drawing pains in the right elbow-joint.

· Drawing pain in the left elbow.

270 · Sharp pains in the arms while in bed, in the morning.

· Rheumatic pains in the right leg and arm.

· Flying, nervous pain, alternating from the left arm to the left eye and parietal region.

· Stitches in the shoulder and hip.

· Wandering pains and soreness in all the limbs.

Lower Extremities.

275 · Aching pains in the back part of the thighs (vv).

· Aching drawing in the left ankle, aggravated by motion, extending up the calf of the leg.

· Rending pains around the left knee; flying, fugitive pains, which come and go rapidly.

· Legs weak, with drawing in the knees and flexor muscles.

· Constant aching distress in the calves of the legs (vv).

280 · Severe, aching distress in the legs all day.

· Hard, aching distress in the right knee all the evening.

· Aching distress in the knees, ankles, and toes.

· Sticking, penetrating pain in the left knee.

· A lame spot on the right knee.

285 · Throbbing pains in the left hip and gluteal region.

· Wandering pains in the limbs and right hip.

· Great weariness of the lower limbs, with trembling (vvvv).

· Drawing pains in the left heel.

Skin.

· A peculiar reddish, clouded appearance of the entire surface of the skin, lasting two days (v).

290 · Red spots on various parts of the body, mostly on the extremities, soon changing to purple, lasting two weeks, with itching around the spots.

· Prickling, like pins, mainly in the popliteal space; itching and burning, like fire; alleviated by sweating.

· Itching and irritation all over, like flea-bites.

· Eruption under the right ear.

· A boil on the forehead. [The prover never had one before.]

295 · A slight bruise inflamed and suppurated.

· Vesicular eruption on various parts; burning and itching, aggravated by exposure to the air.

· Profuse night-sweats.

· Hot skin, *with* profuse perspiration on the forehead.

· Dry heat over the whole body, especially the palms of the hands and the face, with a feeling as if the prover had been up all night; feeling worse when the pains are worse.

Sleep.

300 · Sleep sound, but haunted by frightful dreams (vv).

· Sleep deep and heavy; awaking with racking frontal headache, aggravated by rolling the eyes upwards.

· The sleep is broken and restless (vvvvv), and disturbed by frightful or annoying dreams.

· Frightful dreams, awaking in a profuse perspiration (v).

· Sleep restless, and disturbed by dreams and by drooling of saliva.

305 · Languid on awaking, and unrefreshed (vvvv).

· Nightmare (v).

· Dreams of fighting; of killing snakes.

· Dreams of seeing soldiers.

· Dreams of food.

310 · Dreams very vivid and lifelike.

· Sleep restless, dream-haunted, with pain in the liver on awaking.

· Sleeplessness almost total, from harassing pain in the back; worse in early morning.

· Excessive inclination to sleep during the day.

· Sleep restless and heavy, with fantastic dreams of practising medicine among Brobdingnagians and Liliputians.

315 · Languid and drowsy by day, with bitter taste in the mouth.

· Sleepiness, though he had felt unusually keen, and had enjoyed the full night's rest previous to taking the large dose (500 gtt.).

· Attacked with a kind of nightmare on being awakened at quarter past nine, P.M.; quite conscious, but unable to stir on account of a pressing weight on the stomach, and whole front of the body.

Fever, Pulse, and Heart.

· Flashes of heat, mingled with chilliness, all day. Pulse 88.

Cold chills running up and down the spine.

320 · Feverish heat, lasting all day, *with* pains in the limbs, and nausea (vv).

· Increase of the nausea after dinner, with heat of the skin, and profuse perspiration on the forehead. Pulse 96, small and hard.

· Hot, dry feeling on the body, with cold feet (v).

· Dry heat over the whole body, with sweat on the forehead.

· Chilliness and shivering over the whole body, in a

warm room; inability to keep warm at the stove (after taking five hundred drops).

325 · Pulse 104, an increase of 32 beats in fifteen minutes.

· Shivering in a warm room, *with* heat of the head; shivering over the legs from the hips downwards.

· Pulse 126, small and thready, seventy minutes after the large dose; shivering, with chattering of the teeth; scarcely comfortable near a large fire; but all the symptoms ameliorated in the open air.

· Shivering and horripilation, with eructations tasting of Ptelea.

· Aching distress in all the joints, with great languor (v).

330 · Very languid and faint, *with* flushed face and feverishness (v).

· Rheumatic, drawing pains in all the joints.

· Pulse 72, weak and fluttering.

· Pulse increased twelve beats, soft and weak.

· Pulse accelerated (vvvv) and intermittent.

335 · Hot and feverish all day (vvvvv).

· Hot breath, which seems to burn the nostrils.

· Hot flashes, *with* pain in the top of the head and in the eyes.

· Profuse night-sweats.

· Pulse slow, strong, and irregular.

Generalities.

340 · A curious malaise, with such oppression and weakness at the stomach as to discourage all attempts at work.

· Great lassitude and weariness, with a disposition to hurry through duties (vvv).

· Extreme weakness of limbs, brain, memory, thought, and will (v), as if from a powerful and all-pervading disease.

· Aching of all the limbs, especially of the flexor muscles.

· A fine, violent agitation of all the muscles of body and limbs.

345 ·Dullness, with weakness in upper limbs, extending to lower.

·Great languor and indifference to duties (vvv).

·Soreness of the whole body.

·Frontal headache during the whole proving.

·Rheumatic, drawing, or wandering pains throughout the body.

350 ·Flighty, nervous pains in different parts of the body.

·Loss of energy (v); languor and depression of spirits (Primary).

·Unusual aches and pains all over the body, especially in the abdomen and head.

·Singing increases the nausea, and aggravates the headache, causing shooting pains from within outwards.

·Soreness and swelling of lymphatic glands under the right ear.

355 ·Great restlessness and despondency.

·Irritability of the sensory nerves.

·An unusual energy to work (secondary).

Conditions.

The symptoms assume the form of a severe bilious attack.

All the symptoms suddenly disappear after eating sour things, as sour grapes, or sour apple-sauce.

All the symptoms are better in the cool, open air (primary).

The thoracic symptoms are worse in the keen air (secondary).

The symptoms are all aggravated in the warm room.

The gastric and hepatic symptoms are aggravated by pressure *after meals*, towards morning, and after eating cheese, rich pudding, butter, or any fatty food; but relieved by motion in the open air.

The nausea is aggravated by lying down, or by noise.

The pains in the head press from within outwards.

The headache is *worse* after eating, or from mental exertion, moving the eyes, noise, walking, going upstairs, stooping, or warmth, or during the night, while in bed; but alleviated in the cool, open air, or by pressure.

Predominantly aggravated in the warm room, after eating fatty food, when lying down, or early in the morning, from noise, or when stooping.

Predominantly alleviated in the cool, open air, when rising from bed, or during continued motion, and by the use of vegetable acids.

Directions. — From above downwards, from within outwards, mainly in the right side, or from right to left.

www.ingramcontent.com/pod-product-compliance
Lightning Source LLC
LaVergne TN
LVHW011120110826
845150LV00008B/2205

* 9 7 8 1 4 2 5 5 0 4 1 4 4 *